Y0-EHD-682

The Allergy Gourmet

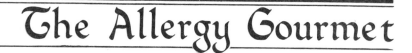

The Allergy Gourmet

by Carol Rudoff, President
American Allergy Association

foreword by William C. Deamer, M.D.
Professor of Pediatrics Emeritus
University of California, San Francisco

illustrations by Brenda Alpinieri

Copyright © 1983 by Carol Rudoff
All rights reserved
Published in the United States by Prologue Publications
First edition

Library of Congress catalog card number: 83—61902
ISBN: 0-930048-11-3

No part of this book may be reproduced
or utilized in any form, electronic or mechanical
including photocopying, recording or any
information storage and retrieval system,
without permission in writing from the publisher.

Inquiries should be addressed to:

Prologue Publications
P.O. Box 640
Menlo Park, CA 94025

To my parents—
their courage, hard work, and continuing love

Contents

Foreword

The diagnosis of food allergy is often, perhaps usually, difficult. This is particularly true with the delayed-in-onset of symptoms type of food allergy as contrasted with the type in which symptoms promptly follow ingestion of the offending food.

Once it has been established that avoiding a certain food (or foods) is beneficial, a patient's problems are usually not over, especially if the offending food was a favorite one. The task of avoiding a food such as milk, wheat, egg, corn and/or chocolate while also avoiding a monotonous menu can become a real problem.

The suggestions Mrs. Rudoff makes in the accompanying recipes will prove helpful in this situation. She obviously knows her way around a kitchen. That the "proof of the pudding is in the eating" finds its application here. Mrs. Rudoff has developed and prepared each of the recipes herself. She has made innovative use of barley flour in replacing wheat and corn, generous use of flavoring with citrus fruits, and employment of a special baking powder and of an egg substitute.

The cookie section will be a welcome one where children and between meal snacks are concerned.

It is a pleasure to recommend this needed addition to the scant literature available to the patient who is told "don't eat it" but is given precious little help in discovering pleasant ways of following such advice.

William C. Deamer, M.D.
Professor of Pediatrics Emeritus
University of California, San Francisco

Preface

Disbelief is the usual response to the allergist's diagnosis of food allergy and disbelief can often be followed by despair. Our feelings of helplessness grow as we note how prevalent milk, eggs, wheat, corn and soy are in our diets. Our traditional recipes as well as the foods we normally buy contain these foods.

What *can* we eat or, worse, how can I take this jigsaw of my family's conflicting food allergies and piece together nutritious and enjoyable meals?

Entertaining becomes a problem. Must we serve two main courses, many different side dishes and two desserts in an effort to meet personal allergy needs and our standards for entertaining guests?

Family dining becomes a problem as we struggle to replace old favorites, try to please various tastes, and attempt to reconcile the different food allergy patterns of different family members.

Even casual entertaining, morning coffee, afternoon tea, children's snacks, Sunday brunch assumes unconquerable proportions.

The Allergy Gourmet presents a series of recipes that you can serve to both family and friends on both casual and festive occasions, recipes that are attractive and nutritious and free from the more common, major allergens.

With *The Allergy Gourmet,* you can entertain at elegant, candlelit dinners and present a dramatic flambe or a sophisticated sauce. These recipes will enable you to serve your family as a family. Family meals should be a time of togetherness, not apartness and struggle. No one should feel isolated and upset at not being able to eat what others are eating. Your family should be able to dine as a unit and you can expect compliments from family and guests alike.

Your doctor's food allergy diagnosis need not result in despair but in hope: now you can do something positive and beneficial for your family's health problems, and with *The Allergy Gourmet*, you can do it triumphantly with flair and culinary style.

C.D.R.

Acknowledgments

I owe special thanks for giving their recipes to be used in this book to Harriet Berner, Marianne Scheck, Jerrell Siegel, Esther Tenenbaum, and Lilyan Zendell.

Thanks is due also to Cathy Zander, home economist, who willingly donated her time to test some of the recipes included here.

To Brenda Alpinieri, close friend of many years, whose beautiful illustrations are the grace notes of this book, I can only and simply say, thank you.

And to my husband, Arnie, and my sons, Neil and Jim, go my deepest appreciation for their patience, support, and philosophical good humor.

Guidelines

Baking without the standard ingredients called for in most recipes is an adventure. Results are subject to the weather, length of storage of ingredients, and a carefully orchestrated balance among the various ingredients.

There are a number of things which influence baking and cooking products and familiarity with these variables will improve your results.

ACCURACY. First check the accuracy of the oven temperature. If you are baking in two ovens, check both since they can differ. Check the accuracy of your timers. They can be off by a surprising amount. Measure carefully. Solid ingredients should be flattened across the tops of the measuring implements. When using a cup to measure liquids, check the liquid level at your eye level.

PAN COLOR AND TIME. If you have dark-colored baking pans, especially the black finish ones, turn the oven temperature down 25 degrees. When baking breads or cakes with these dark pans, lower the temperature of the oven and set the timer for as much as ten minutes less than indicated on the recipe and check frequently for doneness. Mark on the recipe your actual baking time for future reference. For baking cookies on dark sheets, set the timer for several minutes less than the recipe calls for and check frequently for doneness. Taste the cookies to be sure they have the color and texture (crunchy or chewy) you are looking for. Mark on the recipe your actual baking time for future reference. When baking two sheets in the same oven, the bottom sheet cookies may brown first and may even burn before the top sheet is ready. Be prepared to remove the bottom sheet first or to switch locations halfway through baking time.

WEATHER. Since flours can lose moisture during the winter, some recipes may require the addition of liquid and some may need more flour. These additions depend upon how the ingredients 'go together.' If the batter is obviously dry, add water. If it is too soft to handle, add more flour. Damp weather affects sugars after cooking, while cold and heat also affect creaming margarine and sugar.

GLUTEN. Wheat flours have gluten in them and some varieties can have as much as 11% gluten. Eighty percent of the wheat's protein content is gluten which is insoluble in water. When water and flour are mixed to make dough, the mixture is held together by the gluten which becomes elastic and resilient. This process creates a network, trapping carbon dioxide gas from the leavening and expanding with the continuation of the leavening reaction, making gluten the key to raised bread products.

Barley, millet and buckwheat flours do not contain enough gluten to make raised breads. Rice flour is gluten free. If you must avoid gluten, use the table of rice flour equivalents provided below. For baking with rice flour, do not use a waxy type of rice flour; it is for sauces.

Monosodium glutamate and hydrolyzed protein have gluten in them so read the labels carefully. Malt also contains gluten.

LEAVENING. Breads that are leavened with yeast expand to a larger bulk, have a closer grain with thinner cell walls and have a fine texture. Since yeast is a mold and since non-wheat flours do not have the gluten necessary to support the rising power of yeast, our recipes are quick breads and are based on a different type of leavening.

The baking powder and baking soda used in quick breads begin to work in the heat of the oven. These breads can be baked directly after mixing, without waiting. (Double-acting baking powder works during mixing and in the oven.) Without wheat gluten to hold a resilient network of cells high and light, and without yeast, the baked products made from the alternative flours have flavors and textures quite different from wheat and yeast products and they are delicious and flavorful in their own right.

BUTTER. Read margarine labels carefully. Although some diet margarines do not contain milk, they will probably contain corn and/or soy (partially hydrogenated vegetable protein). We have not been able to find a margarine free of milk, corn and soy. If you are sensitive to all three, and if your doctor approves, you may wish to use butter in your baking rather than margarine. Under these circumstances, both Dr. Deamer of the University of California and author of the foreword, and Dr. Vincent Marinkovich, Clinical Associate Professor at Stanford University, permit the use of butter as it is low in the proteins that usually cause allergy problems and is corn-free and soy-free.

In some recipes, you may find you will be able to substitute an equal amount of butter or safflower oil for the melted shortening (usually contains soy) called for. If solid shortening is called for, you can substittue 1 cup of butter or 3/4 cup safflower oil for 1 cup of solid shortening. If you wish to try to substitute for butter, you may try reducing the amount called for by 20 to 25 percent and using safflower oil. We suggest you move cautiously, as these allergen-free recipes have been developed with a fine balance and further substitutions may prove disastrous. The substitutions mentioned in this paragraph should be tried on simple recipes and not complex baked products where relationships among ingredients are very important.

GRAINS. The following are all cereal grains and members of the grass family: wheat, corn (maize), oats, rye, rice, barley and millet.

Barley has a good flavor and is a fine basic flour for baked goods. It is flexible enough to be used in cooking as well. The recipes in this book are based on barley. If you wish to use other flours, you may experiement using the equivalents recommended below.

Buckwheat is not a grain and is not related to wheat. It is a member of the rhubarb family.

Millet is a grain. It can be added to breads and can also be cooked as a breakfast cereal. It is high in B vitamins and iron as well as protein and potassium.

When husked whole kernels of oats are heated and flattened, the results are rolled oats. Rolled oats lack gluten and are grainy. They are better used in combination with other flours and the final product improves if allowed to set before baking.

Rice is grainy and sweet and an excellent flour on which to base recipes; in fact, some may even taste better with rice flour. It is gluten free. Rice and potato starch are a good combination.

Rye is a cereal grass.

If you must avoid wheat, avoid products listing flour, whole wheat, cracked wheat, graham, gluten and monosodium glutamate. Read the labels for bottled sauces as they may contain wheat.

WHEAT EQUIVALENTS:

1 cup of wheat flour equals

1 cup rye meal
1 to 1/4 cups rye flour
1 cup potato flour
1 1/3 cups rolled oats or oat flour
1/2 cup potato flour plus 1/2 cup rye flour
5/8 cup potato starch flour
5/8 cup rice plus 1/3 cup rye flour

BARLEY AND RICE EQUIVALENTS:

1 cup barley flour is equivalent to	1 cup rice flour less 2 tablespoons rice flour
1 1/4 cups is equivalent to	1 1/4 cups less 3 1/2 tablespoons
1 1/3 cups	1 1/4 cups plus 1 tablespoon
1 1/2 cups	1 1/3 cups less 2 tablespoons
1 2/3 cups	1 1/2 cups plus 2 1/3 tablespoons
1 3/4 cups	1 1/2 cups
2 cups is equivalent to	1 3/4 cups
2 1/4 cups	2 cups
2 1/3 cups	2 cups plus 2 1/2 teaspoons
2 1/2 cups	2 1/4 cups less 1 tablespoon
3 cups is equivalent to	2 2/3 cups less 1 tablespoon

DISCUSSION OF INGREDIENTS AND LABELING

MILK. Reading labels should become a habit. You should periodically check the labels even on products you buy frequently, as their contents may change. Many labels will not read 'milk' when they contain milk derivatives. When you see the following words on a label, you should know that they refer to milk products: casein, curds, lactalbumen, lactoglobulin, lactose, sodium caseinate and whey. Several "nondairy" creamers contain sodium caseinate which is derived from milk; these creamers are actually dairy products.

Kosher products (in specialty food section of supermarkets) marked "pareve" do not contain milk, but read their labels as they may contain other foods you are allergic to.

EGGS. Anything with the word 'ovo' in it is an egg ingredient. Egg may appear as powdered egg or dried egg. A substitution for egg you may wish to experiment with is 1 teaspoon (or more) wheat-free baking powder for each egg omitted.

SUGARS. Turbinado is partially refined, coarse brown sugar with a molasses flavor. Brown sugar is made from sugar cane or beets and has molasses added for a brown shade.

Granulated sugar is derived from either beets or cane and is 99.5% sucrose. Some sugars now available are a combination of sucrose with dextrose added in order to attract moisture to the baked product.

Liquid sugars have different sweetening abilities and a higher moisture content than non-liquid sugars; they, therefore, increase the moisture content of the baked product.

Confectioner's or powdered sugar has a small amount of cornstarch added in order to lessen lumping. If you are very corn sensitive, do not use this sugar over cakes or in frostings. Do not substitute for granulated sugar in baking.

Corn syrup is a mixture of dextrose and glucose. If a label mentions dextrose, corn oil, germ meal, gluten meal, corn syrup, caramel or dextrose, the derivative is corn. Fructose syrup on a label may also indicate a corn derivative.

Honey is another sugar and is recognized and digested by the body as a sugar. It contains two sugars: levulose and dextrose. Some honeys may have glucose added. Honey is sweeter than sugar and is semi-liquid, so using it in a recipe calls for some changes. Warming honey in some hot water before measuring it makes it easier to measure. Cakes and cookies made with honey will have a little coarser texture and will be moist and soft.

Honey substitution formlas are:

1. Decrease the amount of sugar by half and use honey in that amount minus 1 tablespoon of liquid less per cup called for in the recipe.

2. Decrease water in the recipe by 1/2 cup for each cup of honey used.

3. For each cup of honey you add, consider it equal to 1 1/4 cups of sugar and decrease the liquid by 1/4 cup and add an extra pinch of baking soda.

4. For every 1/3 cup of white sugar or every 1/2 cup of brown sugar you wish to substitute for, use an extra 1/2 cup flour, 3/4 cup honey and 1/2 teaspoon baking soda.

With so many honey substitution formulas available, it is clear that your choice depends on your taste.

CAROB. Carob is a sweet, high protein, low fat bean, the same color as cocoa with an interesting flavor that is enjoyable in its own right. It is caffeine free and not expensive. With the approval of your doctor, it makes an excellent substitute for chocolate.

Carob powder is available in most health food stores and can be used on an equal basis to replace cocoa in a recipe. Oven temperature should be lowered 25 degrees before baking. If you decide to *add* carob rather than use it as a substitute, remember that it is sweeter than sugar.

Carob Variations are:

1. If you wish to make carob syrup, sift 1 cup of carob powder and add 1 cup of water. Blend, boil and then stir over low heat. Cool until syrup is smooth and store, covered, in the refrigerator.

2. As a substitute for melted chocolate, use 1/2 cup of syrup for every 2 squares of melted bitter chocolate.

3. A second substitute for melted chocolate is to take 1/4 cup of the carob syrup recipe and add 2 tablespoons honey plus 1 tablespoon butter; this can be substituted for 1/3 cup melted semi-sweet chocolate.

4. Semi-sweet carob syrup may be made by adding 1/4 cup honey plus 1 tablespoon butter to the carob powder-water mixture before simmering.

5. If you are unable to find commercial carob chips without milk products in them, use the recipe for carob syrup. Spread the syrup thinly on a paper plate and freeze it. You can then break the frozen carob into chips for use in carob chip cookies.

BAKING POWDER. To substitute for 1 teaspoon of baking powder, try 1/2 teaspoon cream of tarter and 1/2 teaspoon baking soda.

THICKENING. For 1 tablespoon of wheat flour, try the following substitutions:

1. 1/2 tablespoon potato flour
2. 1/2 tablespoon potato starch flour
3. 1/2 to 1 tablespoon arrowroot
4. 1/2 to 1 tablespoon rice flour
5. 2 teaspoons quick cooking tapioca
6. 1 tablespoon tapioca

WATER. Where we have used water in baked recipes (not the water with the egg substitute), you may want to experiment by substituting with fruit juices: orange, apple, pineapple, apricot or grape for flavor variation and for added nutrition.

PRODUCTS. Various products have been used in these recipes. The commercially available egg substitute used was Jolly Joan or Ener G, available in health food stores. Substitutes such as Eggbeaters or Scramblers eliminate only egg yolk (cholesterol). They contain egg whites, casein and milk.

The coconut milk used was Select Coconut Milk (Lorenzana Food Corporation, Philippines) and BKM Coconut Milk (Thai Food Processing, Los Angeles, CA).

Featherweight Baking Powder, cereal-free and available in health food stores, is manufactured by Chicago Dietetic Supply, Inc. of LaGrange, IL.

Carob suppliers are El Molino Mills, Box 2250, City of Industry, CA 91746 and Burry Health Foods Supply, Inc., 43 Reading Blvd., Belle Mead, NJ 08502.

Soy-free seasoning and broth packets, golden and rich brown, are G. Washington's, made by American Home Foods, Inc. New York, NY 10017.

Please check all products before using because ingredients are always subject to change.

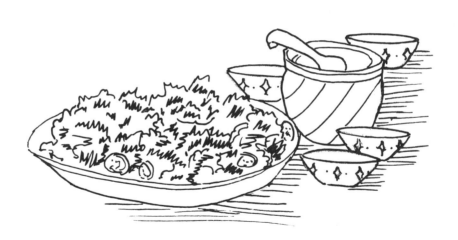

Basic Beef Stock - Marianne

2-3 pounds of English short ribs
  or any beef cut with bones
  (You may also add soup bones.)
2 yellow onions, peeled and quartered
2-3 carrots,
  cleaned and sliced cross-wise
2-3 celery sticks, sliced cross-wise
1 tablespoon parsley
1 bay leaf
1/2 teaspoon chervil
1/2 teaspoon marjoram
1/4 teaspoon salt

Our thanks to Marianne Scheck for the following beef stock and for the three delicious soups (recipes follow) that can be made from it—surely a bit of gourmet magic.

Place ingredients in a soup kettle with water to cover. Simmer for 2 to 3 hours or until meat is tender.

Remove the meat, wrap in aluminum foil and place in refrigerator. Strain stock and place in refrigerator. The next morning remove all surface fat from stock and meat. Cut meat into bite-size pieces. The stock is now ready as a base for the next 3 soups.

VARIATION: BASIC CHICKEN STOCK.. Mrs. Scheck notes that chicken soup stock may be prepared using the beef stock guidelines by substituting chicken for the beef and rice for the barley.

Beef Barley Soup —Marianne Scheck

1 (12 oz.) package pearl barley
1/2 pound fresh mushrooms, sliced
  or canned mushrooms,
  or a combination
  meat from the beef stock recipe
  beef stock from beef stock recipe

Rinse the pearl barley and simmer for 1 hour or until tender in 2 quarts of salted water according to the directions on the package. Strain.

Add the mushrooms, the meat from the beef stock and the cooked barley to the previously prepared stock and simmer for at least 10 minutes. Makes 6 to 8 servings.

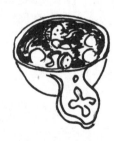

1 pound beets
1 head cabbage, shredded
3-4 medium potatoes,
  peeled and cubed
  meat from the beef stock recipe

Cut the tops from the beets, leaving about 2 inches of stem. Wash the beets and cover them partly with boiling water. Cook, covered, for 30 to 40 minutes if beets are young and up to 2 hours for old beets. Add boiling water if needed. When the beets can be easily pierced by a fork, cool them and slip off the skins. Slice.

Add the beets, the cabbage, potatoes, and cut up meat pieces to the beef stock. Simmer until all vegetables are cooked. Makes 4 to 6 servings.

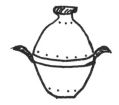

Minestrone —Marianne Scheck

beef stock from beef stock recipe
2-3 medium potatoes,
   peeled and cubed
   carrots or
   zucchini or
   asparagus or
   mushrooms
   meat from beef stock recipe

Add to the beef stock any combination of the above vegetables (or any other allowed vegetables you may have on hand.) Stir in the cut-up pieces of meat from the beef stock preparation and simmer until all vegetables are cooked. Makes 6 to 8 servings.

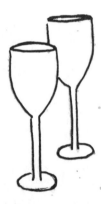

Mushroom Souper

1 pound barley
2 ounces dried mushrooms
24 cups water
1 pound fresh mushrooms
4 tablespoons milk-free margarine

(Barley for soup comes in a cellophane packet; don't use flour.)

Place the barley, dried mushrooms and water in a large soup pot. Bring to a boil and then simmer for 2 hours.

Halve or quarter the larger fresh mushrooms and leave the smaller ones whole. Add the mushrooms to the soup.

Simmer another hour. Just before serving, add the margarine and stir. Makes 12 servings.

Carrot Soup

1/4 cup milk-free margarine
1/2 cup chopped celery
1/2 cup chopped onion
2 tablespoons barley flour
1 1/2 cups chicken stock
2 cups cooked carrots
1 cup water
1/2 teaspoon thyme
1/2 teaspoon tarragon
1/2 teaspoon sweet basil

In the milk-free margarine, saute the celery and onions until limp. Stir in flour and chicken stock. Keep stirring until smooth.

Add the carrots and stir to mix.

Pour the mixture into the blender with water and blend until smooth. Add the seasonings and stir.

Chill and serve cold. Makes 4 to 6 servings.

VARIATION: PUMPKIN SOUP. Substitute a 1-pound can of pumpkin for the carrots.

8 large, ripe tomatoes,
   peeled, seeded and cut up
1 large cucumber,
   peeled, seeded and cut up
1 yellow onion,
   peeled and quartered
1 large green pepper
   seeded and cut up
   salt and pepper to taste
1/4 cup red wine vinegar
1/4 cup olive oil

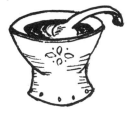

(If you have mold allergy, please check with your doctor before using red wine vinegar. At the 1981 American Academy of Allergy meeting, Dr. W. Busse noted that there is no mention in the literature regarding allergy to olive oil. If you have any questions regarding your own sensitivities, see your allergist.)

Our thanks to Jerrell Siegel for supplying us with this delightfully refreshing cold soup that's deceptively simple to prepare.

Combine the tomatoes, cucumber, onion and pepper in a blender. Add the salt and pepper, red wine vinegar and olive oil.

Place, covered, in the refrigerator for at least 24 hours. Serve over ice cubes. Makes 4 servings.

Cauliflower Soup

1/4 cup milk-free margarine, melted
1 tablespoon arrowroot
1/4 teaspoon nutmeg
1/4 teaspoon cinnamon
3 cups chicken stock
1 small head cauliflower,
  broken into flowerets
1 tablespoon chopped parsley

Place a 10x16-inch oven cooking bag in a 8x12x2-inch baking dish.

Blend the milk-free margarine, arrowroot, nutmeg and cinnamon in a bowl, gradually stirring in the chicken stock.

Pour into bag and add cauliflower. Close bag with a twist tie and make several half-inch slits in the top of the bag near the tie.

Place in a 325° oven for 45 to 50 minutes. Serve with a sprinkling of chopped parsley. Makes 4 to 5 servings.

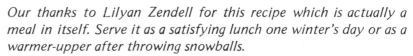

Lilyan Zendell— Meatball Soup

3 cups water
3 cups beef stock
3 potatoes, peeled and cut
3 stalks celery, sliced
3 carrots, peeled and sliced, lengthwise
1 cup instant rice
1 small onion, peeled
1 pound ground beef

Our thanks to Lilyan Zendell for this recipe which is actually a meal in itself. Serve it as a satisfying lunch one winter's day or as a warmer-upper after throwing snowballs.

Heat the 3 cups of water and 3 cups of beef stock in a large soup pot. (While the water is heating, you can peel and cut the potatoes, slice the celery and peel and slice the carrots.)

As water rises to simmer, drop in the potatoes, celery, carrots, rice, and onion.

From the ground beef, form small, half-inch meatballs and toss them into the pot.

When the soup boils, lower temperature to a simmer and continue simmering for 45 minutes. Makes 4 to 6 servings.

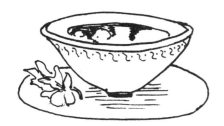

Wild Rice Soup

1/4 cup milk-free margarine
1 medium onion, finely chopped
1/2 pound sliced mushrooms
1/2 cup thinly sliced celery
1/2 cup barley flour
6 cups chicken stock
2 cups cooked wild rice
1/2 teaspoon salt
1/2 teaspoon chervil
1/2 teaspoon basil
1/2 teaspoon marjoram
2 cups coconut milk
1/2 cup dry sherry or madeira
   chopped parsley or chives

No time to cook wild rice? This soup is delicious without it.

Melt the margarine over medium heat in a large saucepan and add the onion. Cook and stir about 5 minutes until the onion is golden.

Add mushrooms and celery and stir for 2 minutes. Slowly mix in flour. Gradually add the broth, stirring constantly until mixture is slightly thickened, about 5 to 8 minutes.

Stir in rice and salt and reduce heat to low. Stir in coconut milk and sherry. Simmer, 5 minutes, stirring occasionally.

Ladle soup into bowls and serve garnished with parsley or chives. Makes 18 servings.

Duck Stock

2 cups chicken broth
1 cup water
  neck and giblets from duck
1/4 teaspoon thyme
1/4 teaspoon tarragon
1 stalk celery, chopped
1 medium onion, chopped

Combine broth and water in a saucepan.

Add neck and giblets, thyme, tarragon, celery and onion. Bring to a boil. Reduce heat to a simmer and cook for 1 1/4 hours.

Avocado Salad

Cut chilled avocados in half and remove the seeds. Fill the hollows with seedless grapes and garnish with mint.

VARIATIONS: Garnish with watercress or parsley; sprinkle raisins over and coconut slivers.

13

Honeydew Salad

1 medium-sized honeydew
1 cucumber
1/2 cup sliced celery
3/4 pound small shrimp
  cooked and shelled
  butter lettuce
2 teaspoons lemon juice
  grated lemon peel
3/4 cup toasted slivered almonds,
  optional

Cut the melon in half and scoop out the seeds. Using a melon ball cutter, scoop the fruit out.

Slice the cucumber thinly and combine with the melon balls, celery and shrimp.

Line a salad bowl with lettuce leaves and spoon in the salad. Sprinkle 2 teaspoons lemon juice and garnish with grated lemon peel. Pass the nuts if you are using them. Makes 4 to 6 servings.

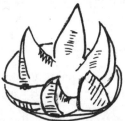

Melon Mold

2 envelopes unflavored gelatin
3/4 cup sugar
1 3/4 cups boiling water
1 cup sherry or madeira
1/4 cup freshly squeezed lime juice
5 cups assorted melon balls,
   Persian, crenshaw, casaba

Combine the gelatin and sugar in a medium bowl. Stir in boiling water, stirring until gelatin is dissolved.

Add sherry and lime juice and mix well.

Chill until the mixture is the consistency of unbeaten egg whites. Then stir in 3 cups of melon balls. Pour into a 5-cup ring mold and chill until firm.

Unmold on a serving plate garnished with the remaining 2 cups of melon balls. Makes 6 servings.

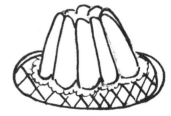

Cranberry Salad

1 tablespoon gelatin
3 tablespoons water
2 cups cranberries
1/2 cup sugar
1/4 teaspoon salt
2/3 cup diced celery

Soak the gelatin in the 3 tablespoons water.

Cook the cranberries until the skins pop in 1 cup of boiling water. Strain the cranberries.

Add to the cranberries the sugar and salt and cook for 5 minutes. Add the soaked gelatin.

Chill. When about to set, add celery . Place in a wet mold and chill until firm. Makes 6 to 8 servings.

Avocado, Mandarin Salad

3 large avocados
1 (16-oz.) can grapefruit segments, drained
1 (11-oz.) can mandarin orange segments, drained
1 small banana, thinly sliced
1/4 cup honey
2 tablespoons lemon juice
  leaf lettuce

Cut avocados in half, lengthwise, and remove pits. Using a teaspoon or melon ball cutter, remove the avocado fruit from the shells. Reserve shells.

Toss avocado with grapefruit segments, orange segments and banana slices.

Mix honey and lemon juice and toss with fruit.

Spoon fruit mixture into avocado shells and place shells on lettuce leaves. Makes 6 servings.

Brunch Pears

3 Bartlett pears
1/2 cup chopped dates
1/2 cup orange juice
1/4 cup honey
2 tablespoons milk-free margarine
   nutmeg

Halve and core the pears; place in a baking dish. Fill the centers with chopped dates.

Combine the juice and honey. Melt the margarine and stir into the juice and honey mixture. Pour over the pears. Sprinkle with nutmeg.

Cover and bake in a 350° oven for 25 minutes, basting occasionally with syrup from the baking dish. Makes 6 servings.

Variation Bananas

Peel and slice bananas on a plate.

HONEY BANANAS. Pour over equal amounts of honey and lime juice.

COCONUT BANANAS. Or. Sprinkle with coconut.

HONEY–CIN BANANAS. Or. Place seedless green grapes over and sprinkle with 1/4 teaspoon cinnamon and 2 teaspoons honey.

STRAWBERRY CIN. Or. Add fresh strawberries and a dash of cinnamon.

ORANGEBERRY CIN. Or. Add fresh strawberries and 1 orange, peeled and sectioned and a dash of cinnamon.

Tomatocado

1 cup tomato puree
  lemon juice
4 cups water
5 avocados, chilled, halved, seeded

Add to the puree, lemon juice to taste and combine with the water.

To still freeze, pour into a refrigerator tray covered with foil and place in freezer. Stir or beat while still slushy. Remove from freezer about 20 minutes before serving. Drop dollops of tomato ice into the avocado hollows. Makes 10 servings.

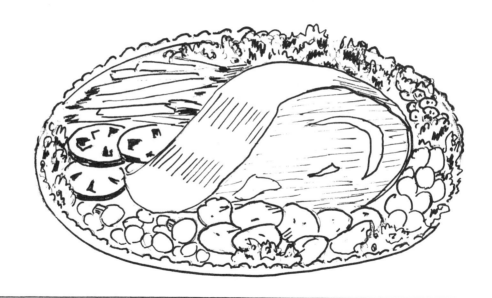

Beef Romanoff

2 tablespoons milk-free margarine
1 pound beef sirloin,
   cut into 1/4-inch strips
3/4 pound sliced mushrooms
3/4 tablespoon grated onion
1 tablespoon milk-free margarine
2 tablespoons barley flour
1 cup cold beef broth
1 cup coconut milk
2 tablespoons dry white wine,
   optional

Our Beef a la Romanoff is especially good served over hot rice or especially traditional served over hot rice noodles.

Melt margarine in skillet or blazer pan of chafing dish. Brown meat strips and add mushrooms and onion. Cook 4 to 5 minutes.

Remove meat and mushrooms. Add margarine and flour. Stir in beef broth. Cook and stir until bubbly.

Return meat and mushrooms to pan. Stir in coconut milk and the wine if you wish. Cook slowly until heated through but do not boil. Makes 4 servings.

Pot Roast

3-4 pound chuck or shoulder roast
   garlic clove, cut
   barley flour
2 tablespoons safflower oil
1 carrot, chopped
1 rib of celery, diced
1 small onion
2 cups boiling meat stock
1 bay leaf
1/4 teaspoon chervil
1/4 teaspoon marjoram

Rub meat with garlic and dredge in flour.

In a heavy oven roasting pan, heat oil and brown meat on all sides. Add remaining ingredients. Cover and bake 3 to 4 hours in a 325° oven or simmer on stove. Turn meat several times and add more stock or water if necessary. When meat is tender, spoon off excess fat, remove bay leaf and serve with sauce. Makes 6 servings.

Beef Stroganoff

1 1/2 pounds fillet of beef
1 tablespoon milk-free margarine
3/4 tablespoon grated onion
2 tablespoons milk-free margarine
3/4 pound mushrooms, sliced
   dash nutmeg
1/2 teaspoon basil
1/4 teaspoon chervil
1/4 cup dry white wine, optional
1 cup coconut milk, warm

Stroganoff is always an elegant company dish and holds well in a chafing dish. Serve over rice or rice noodles.

Cut fillet into 1/2-inch slices across the grain and pound until thin.

Melt the 1 tablespoon of margarine in a pan and saute the onions until golden. Add beef and saute until evenly browned. Remove beef. Add to saute pan the 2 tablespoons margarine and saute the mushrooms. Return beef to pan and season with a dash of nutmeg, basil and chervil. Add wine and warm. Add coconut milk and serve. Makes 4 servings.

Tenderloin of Beef

Serve with broiled mushrooms. Garnish with parsley sprigs.

Preheat oven to 500°.

Trim fat and skin from a 5-pound fillet of beef. Fold over the thin end of the fillet and secure with string.

Spread the meat generously with milk-free margarine or tie strips of bacon over it.

Place on a rack in a roasting pan. Immediately reduce the heat to 400° and bake for 30 minutes. Thermometer should read 130° for rare. Makes 15 servings.

Brisket

3 1/2 pounds brisket of beef
  barley flour
3 tablespoons safflower oil
1 clove garlic, minced
1 teaspoon paprika
  pepper
2 medium onions, sliced
1/2 cup water
2 tablespoons barley flour
1 cup water

If a busy afternoon is on your agenda, you can make this brisket ahead of time and reheat it.

Dredge brisket in flour; brown in oil on high heat. Season to taste with garlic, paprika and pepper.

Place meat in heavy pot. Cover with onions and add water. Bake, covered, until tender in a 325° oven, about 3 hours.

Remove meat from pot and keep warm. Remove all but about 2 tablespoons of fat from the liquid in the pot. Add flour to the drippings and blend. Add water and cook on medium heat until thickened; stir often. Makes 8 servings.

Beef Casserole Brandy

2 pounds beef stewing meat
1 teaspoon paprika
1/2 teaspoon basil
1/4 teaspoon thyme
2 tablespoons barley flour
1 tablespoon safflower oil
1 large onion
2 ounces brandy, optional
10 1/2 ounces beef broth
2 cups sliced fresh mushrooms

Shake the meat together with the seasonings and barley flour until well coated.

Brown the meat slowly in the safflower oil in a heavy skillet.

Cut the onion in wedges and add to the meat. Stir in the brandy and beef broth. Cover tighly and simmer for 1 1/2 to 2 hours until beef is tender.

Add mushrooms for the last 5 minutes. Makes 4 to 5 servings.

Country Time Stew

1 1/2 to 2 pounds beef stew meat
2 teaspoons salt
1 stalk celery, sliced
2 medium onions, quartered
1 bay leaf
4 cups water
4 potatoes, peeled and quartered
6 carrots, peeled and sliced
   or substitute peas or beans
1 cup whole, fresh mushrooms
2 tablespoons barley flour, optional
1/4 cup water, optional

Pressed for time? You can prepare in advance and refrigerate for a day or so or freeze after simmering the beef and removing the bay leaf. If you freeze the beef, thaw it, add the remaining ingredients and continue with the recipe.

Place beef in a large frying pan or Dutch oven. Sprinkle salt over the beef and add the celery, onions, bay leaf and water. Cover and simmer 1 1/2 hours until the beef is tender. Remove the bay leaf.

Add potatoes, carrots (or peas or beans) and mushrooms. Cover and continue cooking until vegetables are tender, 30 to 45 minutes.

If you wish to thicken the liquid, combine the 2 tablespoons barley with the 1/4 cup water and add to the cooking liquid. Cook until mixture boils and thickens. Makes 5 to 6 servings.

Carrot Burgers

1 1/2 pounds ground beef
3/4 cup shredded carrots
1 medium onion, finely chopped
1 teaspoon egg substitute
  plus 2 tablespoons water
1/4 teaspoon chevril
1/4 teaspoon tarragon
1/4 cup rice or barley cereal,
  finely ground

In a large bowl, combine the beef, carrots, onion, egg substitute and water, spices, and cereal crumbs. Shape into 6 patties, about 3/4 inch thick.

Barbecue above glowing coals or broil 3 inches below heat according to your preference. Makes 6 servings.

Sweet 'n Sour Meatballs

1 pound ground beef
2 tablespoons safflower oil
1/4 onion, chopped
1 carrot, grated
2 tablespoons vinegar
1 tablespoon brown sugar
1 teaspoon sherry or marsala wine,
1 tablespoon arrowroot
1/2 cup beef broth
  optional

You'll be surprised at the delicious, special-occasion flavor of this recipe; yet it's so fast and easy, you'll use it frequently.

Form beef into 1-inch meatballs and brown in oil.

Combine onion, carrot, vinegar, brown sugar, sherry and arrowroot. Stir together and add to meatballs along with beef broth. Stir to combine and cook until sauce thickens. Continue cooking for 5 minutes. Makes 4 servings.

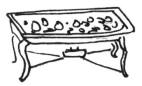

Pan Gravy--Meat

2 tablespoons drippings
2 tablespoons barley flour
  degreased pan juices
  water or wine
  salt, pepper
  herbs
  grated lemon rind

Blend into the drippings. the 2 tablespoons of barley flour and stir until the mixture has thickened and is smooth.

Cook slowly continuing to stir while adding enough of the pan juices, water or wine to make 1 cup. Stir in the seasonings. Makes 1 cup.

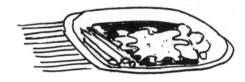

Veal Flambe

2 pounds boneless veal cutlets,
   1/3-inch thick
   salt and pepper
   paprika
3 tablespoons milk-free margarine
2 tablespoons chopped green onions
3 tablespoons barley flour
1 cup coconut milk
1/2 cup dry white wine, optional
1/4 cup brandy or cognac, optional

A spectacular dish (even a make-ahead one) for company. You can also substitute boneless chicken for the veal if you wish.

Trim fat from veal. Pound veal between two pieces of waxed paper with a smooth-surfaced mallet to about 1/4-inch thickness. Sprinkle veal with salt, pepper, and paprika and then cut into 1/4-inch strips.

In a large frying pan, heat margarine over low heat until bubbly. Add green onions and saute. Increase to medium-high heat and cook veal strips, stirring frequently until the veal is no longer pink, about 4 minutes. Remove veal and onions to a bowl.

Stir barley flour into pan drippings and cook, stirring until bubbly. Gradually blend in coconut milk and wine. Cook, stirring until sauce is thickened and smooth.

At this point, you can cover and refrigerate the meat and the sauce separately. Shortly before serving, add cooked meat to hot or reheated sauce in a serving dish. Cook, stirring frequently about 5 minutes or until heated through.

Return veal and green onions to sauce and stir. Heat brandy in a small pan, ignite and pour over veal in sauce. Stir while flaming and then serve. Makes 6 servings.

Veal Compagna

1 1/2 pounds veal cutlets,
   pounded thin
   barley flour
1/4 cup milk-free margarine
1/2 cup chicken broth
   or 1/4 cup chicken broth
   and 1/4 cup Marsala wine
1/2 pound sauteed mushrooms

Dredge veal on one side in flour. Saute, flour side first, in margarine for approximately 3 minutes. Turn and saute other side for 3 minutes.

Remove veal from skillet and keep warm. Add the chicken broth or the broth and Marsala combination. Stir in the mushrooms. Pour over cutlets and serve. Makes 4 to 5 servings.

Veal Scallopini

1 pound boneless veal cutlet
1/4 cup rice flour
2 tablespoons olive oil
  or safflower oil
1/4 cup sauteed mushrooms
1/8 teaspoon nutmeg
1/4 teaspoon marjoram
1 cup chicken broth
1/3 cup white wine or sherry,
  optional
3/4 teaspoon rice flour
1 tablespoon milk-free margarine

Perfect with rice or rice noodles and a crisp, green salad.

Cut veal into strips and pound between two pieces of waxed paper with a smooth-surfaced mallet. Season to taste. Dredge veal in flour and brown slowly in a saucepan with olive oil. Add mushrooms, nutmeg and marjoram. Pour in broth and wine. Simmer for 1 to 1 1/2 hours. Remove veal from saucepan.

Heat together the 3/4 teaspoon rice flour and the margarine and add to liquid in saucepan. Stir and heat.

Return veal to saucepan stir together. Makes 4 servings.

Lamb Francais

2 pounds cubed lamb
1/4 cup olive oil
  or safflower oil
1 clove garlic, minced
  salt and pepper
1/2 teaspoon rosemary
1/2 teaspoon sage
1/2 teaspoon tarragon
1 teaspoon barley flour
1/2 cup white wine
1/2 cup white wine vinegar
  (1/4 cup beef broth,
  if necessary of prevent sticking)

Brown meat in hot oil over high heat, stirring frequently. Add garlic, salt, pepper, rosemary, sage, tarragon and flour, stirring until blended. Heat for 1 minute. Add wine and vinegar and stir again.

Cover pan and simmer for about 45 minutes until meat is tender. Stir from time to time to prevent sticking. (If necessary, add a little beef broth to prevent sticking.) Makes 4 servings.

Festive Leg o' Lamb

6 to 9 pounds leg of lamb
1/3 cup strawberry jam
   (corn-free recipe below)
1/2 teaspoon grated lemon peel
1 tablespoon lemon juice
   dash lime juice
1/4 teaspoon ground ginger
1/2 teaspoon dry mustard
1/4 teaspoon ground pepper

Place lamb on rack in shallow baking pan in a 325º oven.

In a small saucepan, combine jelly, lemon peel and juice, lime juice and spices. Cook and stir over low heat until jelly is melted and the spices are blended.

Brush the lamb with the jelly glaze and continue roasting for 20 to 25 minutes per pound. A meat thermometer should read 140º for rare, 160º for medium or 170º for well done.

In the last hour before the lamb is done, brush about 3 times with the jelly glaze. Makes 8 to 10 servings.

STRAWBERRY JAM: In a medium saucepan, combine 4 cups sliced strawberries, 1/3 cup sugar and 2 tablespoons lemon juice. Heat 5 minutes, crushing berries slightly then bring to a boil. Boil rapidly, stirring constantly, for 3 minutes. In a small bowl, sprinkle unflavored gelatine over cold water and let stand for 1 minute.

Add to strawberry mixture and heat until gelatine is dissolved, about 3 minutes, while stirring constantly. Let the jam stand for 5 minutes and skim off the foam. Ladle the jam into jars. Cover them and cool slightly before refrigerating. For lamb glaze, strain jam before using in recipe.

Honey-Lime Lamb Roast

2 lamb rib roasts
  with backbones loosened
  (3 to 4 pounds)
3/4 cup honey
2 teaspoons grated lime peel
1/3 cup lime juice
1/2 teaspoon parsley
1/2 teaspoon chervil

Place roast, rib side down, in roasting pan. Roast at 325° for 1 hour or until meat thermometer reads 180°.

Meanwhile, heat honey and remaining ingredients in saucepan. During the last 30 minutes of roasting time, baste meat with glaze. Makes 6 to 8 servings.

Herbed Lamb Chops

4 shoulder lamb chops,
   3/4 to 1 inch thick
1/2 teaspoon rosemary
1/2 teaspoon marjoram

Slash outer edge of fat on lamb chops diagonally at 1-inch intervals. Place chops on broiler rack of oven.

Sprinkle with rosemary and marjoram.

Broil chops about 6 minutes on each side. If you wish, season with salt and pepper after broiling. Makes 3 to 4 servings.

Garlic Lamb Chops

4 shoulder lamb chops,
   3/4 to 1 inch thick
  safflower oil
  vinegar
  garlic salt

Slash outer edge of fat on lamb chops diagonally at 1-inch intervals. Brush on each side with oil, vinegar, and garlic salt.

Place chops on broiler rack of oven. Broil about 6 minutes on each side. Makes 3 to 4 servings.

Oranged Lamb Chops

6 shoulder lamb chops,
  3/4 inch thick
1/2 teaspoon shredded orange peel
1/4 cup orange juice
1/2 teaspoon thyme
1/2 teaspoon chervil
1/4 teaspoon marjoram
2 tablespoons safflower oil
1/2 cup sliced mushrooms

Trim excess fat from chops.

Combine orange peel, juice, thyme, chervil and marjoram and spoon over chops. Let stand for 1 hour at room temperature or for several hours in the refrigerator, turning chops over once or twice. Drain, reserving orange mixture.

Brown chops on both sides in hot oil and add orange mixture and mushrooms. Cover and simmer for 40 minutes. Uncover and simmer 5 minutes more. Makes 4 to 6 servings.

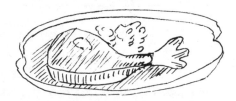

Herbed Lamb Roll

1 tablespoon barley flour
2 teaspoons salt
1 clove garlic, minced
1 tablespoon lemon juice
1/2 teaspoon chervil
1 3 to 4-pound boned and rolled
   lamb shoulder roast
3 tablespoons barley flour

Combine the 1 tablespoon of barley flour, salt, garlic, lemon juice and chervil. Spread over meat.

Enfold the roll securely with heavy foil wrap. Place in a shallow roasting pan in a 425° oven for about 3 hours. Thermometer will register 175° to 180° when ready. Open foil during the last 30 minutes of roasting. Place roast on a warm serving platter.

Pour roasting juices into a 2-cup measuring cup. Add water to make 1 3/4 cups liquid and pour into saucepan. Combine the 3 tablespoons flour with 1/2 cup of cold water and stir into the pan juices. Cook and stir until thick and bubbly. Season to taste. Makes 6 to 8 servings.

Lamb Shoulder Roast

4-5 pound cushion shoulder of lamb
  garlic clove, cut
  dressing for stuffing

Use your favorite, allowed dressing or try our Tangerine Rice Dressing and find a new favorite.

Cut a pocket in one side of the lamb shoulder. Rub the meat with the garlic and stuff with dressing. Skewer closed.

Place roast, uncovered, on a rack in a preheated 450° oven and immediately reduce the heat to 325°. Cook about 30 minutes per pound. Makes 8 servings.

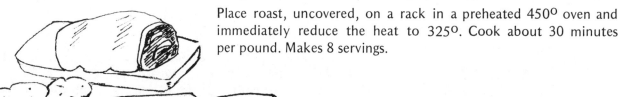

Gingered Pork Crown

1 4 to 5-pound crown roast of pork
1/2 cup pineapple juice
2 teaspoons ginger
2 tablespoons light molasses

Insert thermometer in loin. Be sure the roast is tied around the loin area as well as near bones.

Place roast in shallow roasting pan, bone ends down. Insert meat thermometer. It should not touch bone or fat.

Roast at 325° for 2 1/4 to 2 3/4 hours.

Meanwhile, combine remaining ingredients and baste roast with the glaze four times during last hour of roasting. Thermometer should read 170° when done. Makes 8 to 10 servings.

Glaze 'n Spice Pork

1 2 to 3-pound smoked
   pork shoulder butt
1 medium onion, sliced
3 whole cloves
1 bay leaf
1 3-inch stick cinnamon
1/2 teaspoon celery seed
1/2 cup brown sugar, packed
1 tablespoon barley flour
1/2 teaspoon dry mustard
1/4 teaspoon lemon juice
2 tablespoons water

Place the pork into a large Dutch oven and cover with water. Add onion, cloves, bay leaf, cinnamon and celery seed. Cover tightly and simmer for 2 hours. Remove meat from liquid.

Place meat on rack in a shallow roasting pan.

Combine the brown sugar, flour, mustard, lemon juice and water. Brush on meat and bake for 20 to 30 minutes in a 350° oven. Makes 6 to 8 servings.

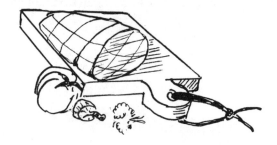

Tangy Pork Chops

2 tablespoons safflower oil
6 pork chops, 3/4-inch thick
1 1/2 cups orange juice
3 tablespoons light brown sugar
1 tablespoon arrowroot
1 1/2 tablespoons grated orange peel
1 1/2 teaspoons salt
1/8 teaspoon ground cloves
3 tablespoons water
2 1/4 tablespoons cider vinegar
1 medium orange, peeled
  and cut into sections
1 medium lime, peeled
  and cut into sections.

Another busy day special because you can make this dish ahead of time and then re-heat it. Serve over rice noodles.

Preheat the oven to 350º.

In a large skillet, heat oil until hot. Brown the pork chops, three at a time, on all sides. Arrange them in a 3-quart baking pan.

Wipe out the skillet with a paper towel and add the remaining ingredients up to and including the cider vinegar. Bring to a boil and pour over the pork chops.

Bake, covered, for 25 minutes and then add the orange and the lime sections. Cook for another 5 minutes or so until the chops are tender. Makes 6 servings.

Pork Chops Pacific

6 loin pork chops, 1/2 inch thick
3/4 teaspoon sage
1/2 teaspoon salt
2 tablespoons safflower oil
2 medium onions, sliced
1 packet brown seasoning and broth
1/4 cup boiling water
1/2 cup coconut milk
1 tablespoon barley flour
2 tablespoons snipped parsley

Rub pork chops with sage and salt. Brown lightly on both sides in oil. Drain off excess fat and add the onions.

Dissolve the seasoning packet in the boiling water and pour over chops. Cover; simmer 30 minutes or until meat is done. Remove to serving platter.

Combine coconut milk and flour in a small bowl then slowly stir the meat drippings into the coconut milk-flour mixture. Return to skillet and cook until boiling while stirring. Add water a little at a time until gravy is of desired consistency. Serve over pork chops and garnish with snipped parsley. Makes 4 to 6 servings.

Pears and Pork Chops

4 to 6 pork chops or steaks
  salt and pepper
3 to 4 fresh pears, halved and cored
2 tablespoons orange juice
1/4 cup packed brown sugar
1/4 teaspoon cinnamon
1/4 cup dry sherry or orange juice
1 tablespoon milk-free margarine
1 teaspoon arrowroot
1 tablespoon water

Grease the bottom of a frying pan with a small piece of pork fat. Brown chops over medium heat, turning once. Place in a shallow pan and sprinkle with salt and pepper. Place pears around the chops and drizzle orange juice over. Sprinkle with brown sugar and cinnamon and then pour the sherry. Divide the margarine and place in the hollow of the pears.

Cover and bake at 350° for 40 minutes. Uncover during the last 20 minutes of baking.

Remove pears and chops to warm serving platter. Dissolve arrrowroot in water. Add to juices in pan and bring to a boil. Sauce will thicken. Pour over chops and pears. Makes 4 to 6 servings.

Pork L'Orange

6 pork chops, 1/2 inch thick
1 teaspoon salt
1 medium onion, cut into 6 slices
1 6-ounce can frozen orange juice
   concentrate, partially thawed
1/4 cup packed brown sugar
1/2 teaspoon allspice
3 tablespoons lemon juice
3/4 cup water
4 baked sweet potatoes,
   peeled and sliced crosswise
   into 1/2-inch slices
6 thin orange slices

Trim excess fat from chops and brown on both sides in a greased, 12-inch skillet. Season with salt and drain fat. Place an onion slice on each chop.

Combine orange juice concentrate, sugar, allspice, lemon juice and water and pour into skillet. Heat to boiling. Reduce heat and cover. Simmer 25 minutes.

Arrange sweet potatoes around the chops and place an orange slice over each onion slice on the chops. Cover and cook 15 minutes longer or until potatoes are heated through. Makes 4 to 6 servings.

Baked Ham Slice L'Orange

1/2 cup packed brown sugar
1 tablespoon arrowroot
1/8 teaspoon ground ginger
1 cup orange juice
1 teaspoon grated orange peel
1 teaspoon lemon juice
1 ham slice, cut 1-inch thick
8 whole cloves

In shallow baking dish, combine brown sugar, arrowroot, and ginger. Stir in orange juice, grated orange peel, lemon juice. Add ham slice, turning to coat both sides. Sprinkle with cloves.

Bake, uncovered, 45 to 60 minutes, in a 325° oven, basting ham occasionally with sauce. Makes 4 to 5 servings.

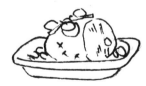

Ham Slices Variety

Place a ham slice, 1-inch thick, in a casserole with a cover. Select one of the recipes below and bake the ham, covered, for 45 minutes at 325° until tender, basting several times with the juices in the pot. Uncover for the last 10 minutes.

I: HAM APPLE OLE. Cover ham with sliced apples. Sprinkle with brown sugar or honey; bake.

II: HAM A LA ORANGE. Cover ham with oranges. Sprinkle with brown sugar or honey; bake.

III: PINEAPPLE HAM. Cover ham with sliced of canned pineapple. Sprinkle with cinnamon; bake.

IV: APRICOT HAM. Cover ham with canned apricot halves and sprinkle with cinnamon, brown sugar. Bake.

V: PEACHY HAM. Cover ham with canned peach slices. Sprinkle with honey, cinnamon. Bake.

VI: CHERRIES HAM. Cover ham with canned cherries (not pie filling). Sprinkle with cinnamon. Bake.

VII: HAM WITH FRUIT JUICE OR SHERRY. Baste with a cup of fruit juice or sherry.

Makes 2 to 3 servings.

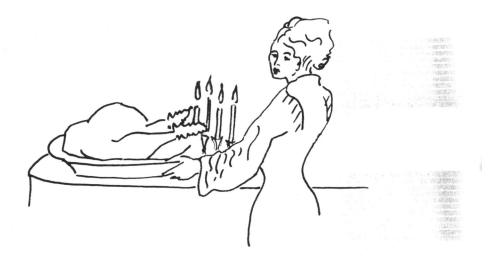

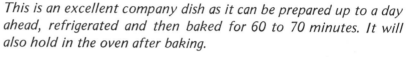

Artichoke Chicken

10 chicken breast halves
  salt, pepper, paprika
4 tablespoons milk-free margarine
1 (15 oz.) can artichoke hearts,
  drained and halved
2 tablespoons milk-free margarine
3/4 pound fresh mushrooms, halved
2 tablespoons barley flour
3 tablespoons sherry, optional
1 to 1/4 cups chicken broth or stock

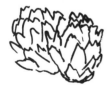

This is an excellent company dish as it can be prepared up to a day ahead, refrigerated and then baked for 60 to 70 minutes. It will also hold in the oven after baking.

Season the chicken and brown in the 4 tablespoons of milk-free margarine. Transfer to a large casserole and scatter the artichokes among the chicken breasts.

Place the 2 tablespoons of milk-free margarine in the skillet and saute the mushrooms for five minutes. Sprinkle flour over and stir in sherry and broth. Stir gently over low heat until mixture thickens. Then pour the mushroom sauce over chicken.

Cover and bake in a 375° oven for 45 minutes. Check about halfway through baking time to see if more broth is needed. Serves 8 to 10.

Chicken Limon

1 3-pound broiler-fryer, cut up
safflower oil
1 tablespoon tarragon
1 tablespoon basil
2 tablespoons milk-free margarine
1 1/2 tablespoons barley flour
3/4 cup chicken broth, boiling
2/3 cup orange juice, heated
1/4 cup Marsala wine, optional
grated peel of 1 lemon

With minimal preparation, you can serve Chicken Limon *to your most sophisticated guests. The flavors blend with exotic subtlety.*

Rub chicken with oil and sprinkle with tarragon and sweet basil. Place chicken in baking dish.

Melt the margarine. Stir the remaining ingredients into the melted margarine and pour this sauce over the chicken.

Bake in a 350° oven for 1 hour. Makes 4 servings.

Chicken Saute Herbed

1 3-pound broiler-fryer, cut up
1/2 stick milk-free margarine
1 tablespoon safflower oil
4 shallots, minced
1 tablespoon lemon juice
1/4 cup dry white wine, optional
1 tablespoon chopped parsley
1 teaspoon tarragon
1/2 teaspoon rosemary
1/4 teaspoon thyme

An excellent chicken saute, with a delicate flavor—perfect for company. The sauce is excellent. Try using it as the liquid for rice.

Brown chicken in margarine and oil and add the shallots. Cook for about 3 minutes.

Sprinkle lemon juice, wine and herbs over the chicken. Cover and cook for 15 minutes.

Turn chicken over. Cook over low heat for 30 minutes, partially covered, until chicken is done. Makes 4 servings.

Apricot Chicken

4 chicken breast halves
8 large, fresh apricots
2 tablespoons grated lime rind,
 optional
2 tablespoons lime juice, optional
2 tablespoons honey

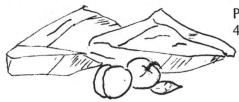

Apricot Chicken *can be made in advance and refrigerated for later heating. It is the perfect supper to leave for the children and sitter or to have prepared when you will be away all day.*

Puree apricots, lime rind, lime juice and honey in a blender.

Cut four large squares of aluminum foil and place a chicken breast on each square. Pour sauce over, dividing among the four squares. Fold the foil over the chicken securely.

Place packets in a baking dish and bake in a 375° oven for 30 to 45 minutes. Serves 4.

Lime Chicken

4 whole chicken breasts,
  skinned and boned
1 small carrot, chopped
1 stalk celery, chopped
1 1/3 cups water
1 packet golden seasoning and broth
2 tablespoons milk-free margarine
2 tablespoons safflower oil
1 medium onion, sliced
1/2 pound mushrooms, sliced
3 tablespoons barley flour
1/4 cup dry vermouth, optional
3 tablespoons lime juice
1 bay leaf
1/4 teaspoon thyme
1/4 teaspoon marjoram
1/4 teaspoon basil
1/4 coconut milk

Place bones and skin in a 3-quart pan with carrot, celery, water and seasoning packet. Cover; bring to a boil and then reduce heat. Simmer 30 to 45 minutes. Pour through a wire strainer and set broth aside. Your yield should be approximately 1 cup.

Heat margarine and oil in a frying pan over medium heat. Brown the chicken breasts until golden. Set the chicken aside.

To pan drippings, add the onion and mushrooms and cook until the onion is limp. Stir in flour. Cook until bubbly and then add vermouth and lime juice, the 1 cup of broth and the spices.

Continue cooking, stirring until the sauce is bubbly and thickened. Stir in the coconut milk and add salt and pepper to taste.

Return chicken to pan. Cover and simmer for 15 minutes or until chicken is opaque when slashed. Remove chicken to serving plate.

Skim fat from sauce; spoon the sauce over the meat. Garnish with chopped parsley. Pass remaining sauce at table. Makes 8 servings.

Vegetable, Chicken Bake

1 clove garlic, crushed, optional
2-3 tablespoons olive oil or safflower
1 2-1/2 to 3 pound chicken, cut up
2 carrots, pared and sliced
  into slender sticks
2 stalks celery, sliced
  into slender sticks
1/2 pound mushrooms, thinly sliced
1/4 cup white wine, optional

Saute garlic in oil. Add chicken and brown. Remove chicken from saucepan.

Cook carrots, celery and mushrooms in saucepan. Pour in wine.

Return chicken to pan.

Bake in a 350° oven for 1 hour or simmer on stove until chicken is tender, about 1 hour.

Add zucchini the last 10 minutes. Makes 4 servings.

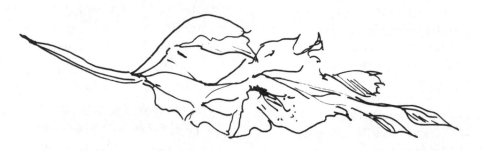

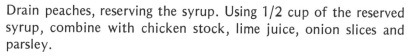

Peach and Lime Chicken

1 can (16 oz.) cling peach halves
1 cup chicken stock
1/2 cup lime juice
1 medium onion, thinly sliced
2 tablespoons snipped parsley
1/8 teaspoon rosemary
1/8 teaspoon thyme
1 3-pound chicken, cut in pieces
1 lime, thinly sliced

Drain peaches, reserving the syrup. Using 1/2 cup of the reserved syrup, combine with chicken stock, lime juice, onion slices and parsley.

Place chicken in dish and pour peach mixture over. Refrigerate for 5 hours or overnight in this peach-lime marinade.

Remove chicken from marinade and broil 6 inches from heat (6 or more minutes per side).

Meanwhile, in a small saucepan, combine peaches, remaining syrup and the peach-lime marinade. Stir over medium heat until well heated.

Arrange chicken on serving plate, surrounded with peach halves. Pour hot sauce over and garnish with lime slices. Makes 4 to 5 servings.

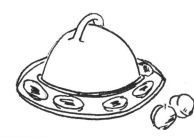

Orange Chicken

1/2 cup barley flour
2 teaspoons grated orange peel
1 teaspoon paprika
3 pounds chicken parts, skinned
1 tablespoon safflower oil
1/2 cup water
1 1/2 cups orange juice
2 tablespoons light brown sugar
3/4 teaspoon ground cinnamon
1/4 teaspoon ground ginger
1/8 teaspoon nutmeg

Combine flour, orange peel and paprika. Measure 2 tablespoons of mixture and set aside. Coat chicken pieces with remaining flour.

In a large skillet, heat oil until hot. Brown the chicken. Add the water and bring to a boil. Reduce heat and simmer, covered, for about 30 minutes or until chicken is tender.

Remove chicken to a serving platter. Stir reserved flour mixture into the skillet. Add remaining ingredients, stirring until thickened. Spoon sauce over chicken. Makes 4 servings.

Poulet Flambe

1 3-4 pound broiler
   safflower oil
2 tablespoons milk-free margarine
   melted
1 tablespoon lemon juice
1/2 teaspoon parsley
1/4 teaspoon tarragon
1 oz. warmed brandy, **optional**

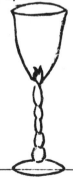

Celebrate your gala events with this delicious and spectacular dish.

Cut chicken into halves or quarters. Rub with oil.

Place the chicken, skin side down, under preheated broiler, at least 5 inches from the heat. Broil chicken until brown, about 15 to 20 minutes for each side.

Combine the melted margarine, lemon juice, parsley and tarragon. Just before turning chicken, baste with this herb mixture. Turn and baste again.

Before serving, be sure brandy is warm. Set flame to the brandy and pour over the chicken. Makes 4 servings.

Chicken in the Pot

2-3 cups cooked chicken,
  cut in chunks
1 can (1 lb.) whole onions
1 can (1 lb.) sliced carrots
  or frozen carrots
  or fresh cooked carrots
1 can (1 lb.) cut up green beans
  or frozen green beans
  or fresh cooked green beans
1/4 cup chicken broth
1/2 teaspoon salt
1/4 teaspoon thyme
1/8 teaspoon marjoram

In 4 1/2-quart kettle, combine chicken, onions with liquid, carrots with liquid, green beans with liquid, chicken broth and seasonings.

Heat to boiling, stirring occasionally. Ladle generous portions into soup bowls. Makes 5-6 servings.

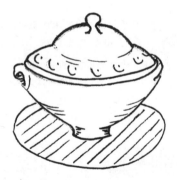

Poulet Marsala

4 tablespoons milk-free margarine
1/2 teaspoon tarragon
1 3-1/2 pound chicken
1/2 cup Marsala wine, optional
1 tablespoon barley flour
3/4 cup chicken stock

Place margarine and tarragon inside cavity of chicken. Place the chicken in a roasting pan. Pour the Marsala over.

Roast in a 375° oven for about 1 1/2 hours, basting often with drippings.

Remove from oven and let liquids pour into roasting pan. Make gravy by adding flour and stock to drippings. Heat and stir until thick and bubbling. Makes 4 servings.

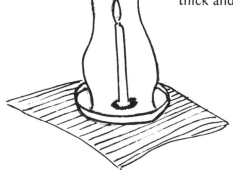

Chicken Breasts Marsala

2 tablespoons milk-free margarine
4 tablespoons olive oil or safflower
4 chicken breasts, halved
1/2 cup chicken stock
1/4 cup Marsala wine, optional
1/4 pound mushrooms, sliced
   chopped parsley

In a large, ovenproof casserole, melt the margarine with the olive oil and brown the chicken breasts. Pour off all but 1 tablespoon of fat.

Add chicken stock and Marsala. Cover and simmer for 30 to 35 minutes. Add mushrooms, cover and cook for 5 minutes longer. Garnish with chopped parsley. Makes 4 servings.

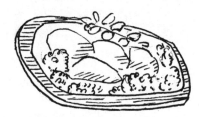

Chicken Pot Pie

DOUGH:
2 cups barley flour
1 teaspoon salt
2/3 cup safflower oil
3 tablespoons cold water

Stir together the flour and salt. Combine the oil and water and quickly pour the oil mixture into the flour all at once. Stir gently with a fork until blended. Place the dough into a pie pan and pat it to fit. Generously prick the sides and bottom and bake in a 475º oven for 12 to 15 minutes. Cool slightly.

Meanwhile, make the filling. An excellent way to serve leftovers. Whatever you have just goes into the pot and don't worry about measuring.

FILLING:
In a saucepan, put 1 cup of chicken broth, approximately 2 cups of cubed, cooked chicken, cooked, cubed vegetables (carrots or broccoli or whatever you have available), boiled potatoes in chunks.

Measure 1 1/2 teaspoons of arrowroot into 1/4 cup of water and mix. Add 2 or 3 tablespoons warm broth to arrowroot and stir. Pour arrowroot into broth. Heat and stir until bubbly and pour into pie shell. Makes 4 servings.

Variety Chicken

2-3 large chicken breasts
2 tablespoons sesame seeds
   safflower oil
1/2 pound mushrooms,
   washed and sliced
1 small green bell pepper, diced
1/2 small clove garlic, pressed
1 packet chicken seasoning
1 cup hot chicken broth
2 tablespoons arrrowroot
2 cups hot cooked rice
   or rice noodles

Remove skin from chicken breasts; slice into small chunks and saute along with sesame seeds in vegetable oil in a large frying pan until chicken turns white.

Add mushrooms, bell pepper and garlic. Continue cooking over medium heat.

Dissolve chicken packet seasoning in hot chicken broth. In a small bowl, blend arrowroot into 3 tablespoons of the chicken broth and stir back into the chicken seasoning and broth mixture. Cook, stirring until sauce thickens slightly.

Spoon chicken and sauce over rice or rice noodles. Makes 6 servings.

4 chicken thighs (1-1 1/4 pounds)
  barley flour
1 tablespoon milk-free margarine
1 tablespoon safflower oil
1/3 cup chicken broth,
  or 1/3 cup dry white wine
1/4 cup coconut milk
1 teaspoon lemon juice
1/4 teaspoon thyme

Here's a gourmet dish on a budget. Present it with a flourish, garnished with parsley sprigs and lemon wedges over rice.

Remove skin from chicken thighs. On the inside of each thigh, cut to the bone along the length of the thigh and scrape the meat free from the bone. Place meat between sheets of waxed paper and pound the meat gently until it is about 1/4-inch thick. Dust the meat with barley flour.

Melt margarine and oil in a large frying pan over medium high heat. Add as many slices of meat as will fit without crowding pan and cook quickly, about 1 1/2 minutes per side. Keep warm on a hot platter.

Add chicken broth or white wine, stirring to blend. Boil until reduced by about half. Add coconut milk, lemon juice, and thyme and boil until sauce thickens slightly.

Juices that have collected on meat platter may be poured into sauce and stirred. Pour over meat and garnish. Makes 2 servings.

Chicken Sherry

1 2 1/2-3 pound broiler-fryer, cut up
2 tablespoons milk-free margarine
1 medium onion,
   chopped and sauteed
1 clove garlic, crushed
1 cup chicken stock
2 stalks celery, sliced and sauteed
2 cups water
1 cup mushrooms,
   sliced and sauteed
1/4 cup sherry, optional

Brown chicken in margarine. Place in ovenproof casserole with onion, garlic, chicken stock, celery and water.

Bake, covered, in a 350° oven for 45 minutes.

Remove cover and add mushrooms and sherry. Continue baking, uncovered, for 15 minutes. Makes 4 servings.

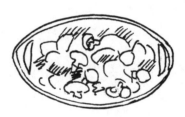

Chicken Elegante

1 3-pound broiler fryer
1 tablespoon lime juice
1 teaspoon grated lime peel
  salt, pepper, paprika
1/4 teaspoon chevril
1/8 teaspoon tarragon
1 1/2 cups seedless grapes
1/3 cup dry white wine
  or chicken broth

Wash chicken and pat dry. Rub with lime juice and sprinkle over with lime peel, salt, pepper, paprika, chevril and tarragon.

Place chicken in a roasting pan and stuff the cavity with grapes. Roast in a 400° oven for 20 minutes. Lower the heat to 325° and continue roasting for 1 to 1/4 hours until drumstick moves easily. Baste several times during roasting period with wine and drippings.

Carve and serve with grapes and pass pan juices with the fat skimmed off. Makes 4 servings.

Pan Gravy--Poultry

1/4 cup fat from a roasted foul
1/4 cup barley flour
  pan juices
  poultry stock
  chopped, cooked giblets

After straining the juices from a roasted foul, pour off and save the fat for gravy. Blend the barley flour into the fat, and then slowly stir in enough of the pan juices and poultry stock to make 2 cups.

Cook and stir the gravy until it is smooth and then simmer for 5 minutes. Add the giblets. Makes 2 cups.

Cornish Game Hen

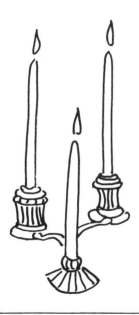

Select a hen about 1 1/2 to 2 pounds and bake in a 375° oven for 45 minutes to 1 hour.

Cornish hens are a good substitute for chicken and most chicken dishes are readily adapted. Simply change the baking time and try any of the preceding poultry recipes in this section.

One hen serves 1 or 2, depending upon appetite.

You can also vary the stuffings and basting for further variety. See the *Potpourri* section for suggestions.

Cornish Game Hen Sauces. 1. Combine 3 tablespoons melted milk-free margarine and 1 tablespoon each of lemon juice, lime juice, orange juice and honey and baste during the last 20 minutes of cooking time. 2. Combine 3 tablespoons melted milk-free margarine and 1 tablespoon each of chervil, marjoram and basil and baste frequently. Check index for other selections.

Turkey Breasts Marsala

1 1/2 pounds turkey breasts
  barley flour
1/4 cup milk-free margarine
1/2 cup chicken stock
3 tablespoons Marsala wine
  or 1 tablespoon lemon juice

Top the breasts with 1/4 pound sliced and sauteed mushrooms and serve over rice.

Dredge the turkey breasts in the flour and saute in the milk-free margarine. Continue cooking over low heat, shaking the pan to prevent the meat from sticking.

When cooked through, add the chicken stock and Marsala. Makes 4 servings.

Turkey Almondine

2-4 tablespoons safflower oil
2 cups diced cooked turkey
1/2 cup diced water chestnuts
1/2 cup diced bamboo shoots
1/2 cup diced celery
1/2 cup sliced mushrooms
2 tablespoons Marsala wine, optional
3/4 cup chicken broth
1/2 teaspoon sugar
2 teaspoons arrowroot
  water
  toasted almond halves

Heat oil in skillet. Add turkey and brown lightly. Remove turkey.

Add water chestnuts, bamboo shoots, celery and mushrooms, cooking and stirring until vegetables are tender, but maintain some crispness. Add Marsala and broth. Cover for about 30 seconds to steam.

Add sugar and the cooked turkey that you have set aside.

Blend arrowroot with water and stir to make a smooth paste. Gradually blend the arrowroot mixture into the skillet and cook, stirring until thickened. Sprinkle with almonds. Makes 4 servings.

Turkey Fricassee

5 pounds of turkey meat, chunked
3 cups water
1 carrot, sliced
2 ribs of celery, with leaves
1 small onion, sliced
1 recipe Pan Gravy—Poultry

Place the turkey pieces in a large pot with 3 cups of water along with the carrot slices, celery and onion slices. Bring to a boil and then reduce to a simmer. After about 15 minutes, remove the scum at the surface and continue to simmer until the meat is tender, 2 hours or more.

Remove the meat and strain the stock. If you prefer very thick gravy, boil the stock to reduce it to 1 1/2 cups before thickening. Thicken with barley flour; see Pan Gravy recipe.

Pour the gravy over the chicken and garnish with parsley. Makes 5 servings.

Duck in Apricot Sauce

1 4-pound duck
2 tablespoons honey
1 (16-oz.) can apricot halves,
   reserve syrup
2 tablespoons lemon juice
   water
1/2 teaspoon grated lemon rind
1 tablespoon arrowroot
1 tablespoon sugar
1 tablespoon milk-free margarine
2 tablespoons apricot brandy,
   optional

Place the duck on a rack in a roasting pan in a preheated 450° oven. Reduce the heat at once to 350° and bake, uncovered, for 1 hour. Brush duck with honey and return to oven until done, allowing 20 minutes per pound total.

Meanwhile, prepare sauce. Using the juice from the can of apricots, add lemon juice and enough water to make 1 cup of liquid.

Pour the apricot-lemon liquid into a saucepan along with the lemon rind, arrowroot, sugar, and margarine. Whisk the sauce while bringing it to a boil and keep whisking until smooth and thickened.

Reduce heat and add apricots and brandy. Heat thoroughly, but don't boil. Serve the duck with the sauce. Makes 4 servings.

Orange Duck Almondine

1 5-pound duckling
1 cup orange marmalade
1/4 cup blanched, slivered almonds,
  optional
2 tablespoons almond liqueur,
  optional
  or curacao, optional
  or 1 tablespoon lemon juice

Serve with a flourish on a carving platter garnished with glazed carrots and almonds surrounded by mounds of wild rice.

Place the duck on a rack in a roasting pan in a preheated 450° oven. Reduce the heat at once to 350°. Allow 20 minutes to the pound for an unstuffed bird. Baste periodically for a crisp skin.

Meanwhile, in a saucepan, combine marmalade, almonds, and liqueur. Simmer for 1 hour over low heat.

Approximately fifteen minutes before the duck is done, drain the grease off and pour the orange sauce over. Leave the duck in the oven for the remaining 15 minutes. Makes 4 to 5 servings.

Duck Continental

1 medium onion, peeled
  and left whole
1 large slice of cooking apple
1 5-pound duck with liver
3 medium onions. peeled
  and quartered
3 carrots, peeled and chopped
1/4 cup red wine, optional
  or 1 tablespoon lemon juice
2 tablespoons milk-free margarine

Place whole onion, apple, and liver inside cavity of duck and close cavity. Prick skin. Place duck, breast side up, on a rack in a roasting pan and surround with the quartered onions and carrots. Place in preheated 450º oven and immediately lower the temperature to 350º and bake, uncovered, until done, allowing about 20 minutes per pound. Remove from oven, discarding onion, apple and liver. Place duck on a serving platter. Makes 4 servings.

SAUCE: Strain the drippings from the roasting platter. Measure 2 cups of the strained duck stock and return to pan, retaining the carrots and onions. Bring to a boil. Mash vegetables. Pour in red wine and simmer a few minutes. Stir in margarine. Simmer gently a moment or two; strain and serve.

Cherried Duck Flambe

1 5-pound duck
3 tablespoons cognac
1/2 cup dry white wine
1/4 cup chicken stock
   pinch cinnamon
1 tablespoon sugar
2 cups Bing cherries, pitted

Place the duck on a rack in a roasting pan, breast side up, in a pre-heated 450° oven. Reduce the heat at once to 350° and bake, un-covered, for approximately 20 minutes per pound.

When duck is done, warm the cognac; ignite it and pour it over the duck. Cut the duck in quarters and place on a heated serving dish.

Using the roasting pan, bring the wine, stock, cinnamon and sugar to a boil. Add the cherries and simmer, covered, for 5 minutes. Pour the cherry sauce over the duck. Makes 4 servings.

Fish

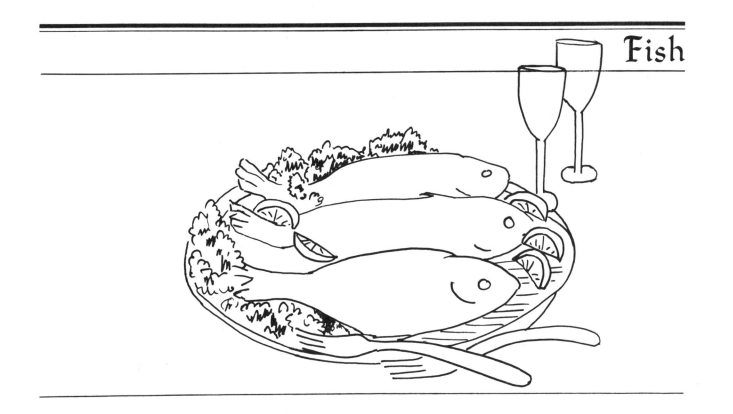

Inserting a thermometer into the thickest part of the flesh is the most accurate way of ascertaining doneness. Fish is done when the temperature measures 140°. At 150°, juices start escaping, so be sure not to let the fish cook beyond 145°. A wooden pick thrust into the thickest part of the flesh, meeting little resistance as it goes in and coming out clean, is a sign of doneness. When the fish is no longer translucent (it becomes opaque) and its flesh flakes when tested with a fork, it is done.

Use pan poaching for delicately flavored fish like flounder, sanddabs, sole, halibut, turbot. Cod, haddock, salmon, trout, whitefish, bass and mullet can also be poached.

PAN POACHING: Rinse and pat dry 2 pounds fillets, steaks, or packaged frozen fish. In a large frying pan, melt 1 tablespoon milk-free margarine. Add 2 green onions, chopped and 1 clove of garlic, pressed. Cook and stir until onions are limp and add 1/2 cup chicken broth. Bring to a boil and place fish in pan. Reduce heat; cover pan; simmer until fish flakes when fork-tested. Makes 4 servings.

Flounder, sanddabs, sole, halibut, turbot, cod, haddock, salmon, trout, whitefish, bass and mullet can be pan fried.

PAN FRYING: Rinse and pat dry 2 pounds fillets, steaks, or packaged frozen fish. Dredge fish in barley flour or dip in water and then in a crumbed rice or barley cereal. Over medium heat, heat safflower oil (about 1/8-inch deep) in a large frying pan and arrange fish in pan. Cook until flesh flakes when fork-tested and then turn over. Makes 4 servings.

Cod, haddock, rockfish, salmon, whitefish, trout, bass and yellowtail can be oven browned.

OVEN BROWNING: Using 2 pounds of fillets, steaks or packaged frozen fish that are 1/2 to 1 inch thick, rinse and pat dry. Melt 3 tablespoons milk-free margarine. Make 1/4 to 1/2 cup of crumbs from rice or barley cereal and mix with 1/4 teaspoon thyme, 1/4 teaspoon paprika, 1/4 teaspoon chervil. Dip the fish in the margarine and then in the crumbs to coat. Place in a foil-lined shallow baking pan and bake, uncovered, in a 425° oven for 15 to 20 minutes for fresh fish and about 30 minutes for frozen fish. Makes 4 servings.

Cod, haddock, rockfish, salmon, whitefish, trout, bass, yellowtail, and mackerel can be foil cooked.

FOIL COOKING: Rinse and pat dry 2 pounds of fillets, steaks, or frozen fish and place them on foil rectangles large enough to enclose them. Sprinkle 2 tablespoons green onion, 1 tablespoon chopped parsley, 1/2 teaspoon chervil, 1/2 teaspoon marjoram and wrap each serving securely with the foil. Place on an oven sheet and bake in a 425° oven, allowing 12 to 15 minutes for each 1 inch of thickness of the fish. Drain liquid after baking. Makes 4 servings.

Cod, pollock, haddock, salmon, trout, whitefish, bass, yellowtail, and mahimahi can be oven baked.

OVEN BAKING: Rinse and pat dry 2 pounds of fillets, steaks, or frozen fish. Lightly grease the fish and set it on an oiled rack in a large baking dish. Place the dish in a preheated 350° oven, slightly higher than the middle of the oven. Turn the fish once, carefully with a spatula. Fish is done when flesh flakes after fork testing. Makes 4 servings.

Turbot in Vino

1 pound turbot fillets
2 tablespoons milk-free margarine
1 clove garlic, crushed
1/4 cup dry white wine
1/2 teaspoon basil
1/4 teaspoon chervil
  paprika, optional
  lemon wedges
  watercress or parsley

If in one piece, cut turbot in half.

Melt the margarine in a skillet. Swish the garlic around the pan and discard. Pour in the wine and heat just to boiling. At this point, add the fish. Cook very briefly, just until flesh starts to flake when fork-tested. Carefully turn the fillets over with a spatula and cook the other side. Sprinkle with basil and chervil; add color with the paprika. Ladle the cooking liquid over the fish and garnish with lemon wedges and watercress or parsley. Makes 2 servings.

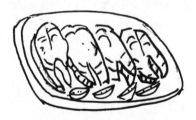

Snapper a la Pear

1 Anjou pear,
   peeled and cut into strips
2 tablespoons fresh lemon juice
1 pound red snapper
   salt
   barley flour or arrowroot
1 tablespoon milk-free margarine
1 tablespoon safflower oil
2 tablespoons milk-free margarine
1/4 cup slivered almonds, optional
1 teaspoon grated lemon peel
1/2 cup seedless green grapes

Marinate pear in lemon juice.

Season fish with salt and dust lightly with flour or arrowroot. In a large skillet, saute fish in margarine and oil until lightly browned on both sides. The flesh will separate when fork-tested. Transfer to a heated platter.

Add the 2 tablespoons of margarine to the pan and heat. Add nuts and toast lightly, constantly stirring. Add lemon peel, grapes, and pears. Heat gently and briefly. Spoon over fish. Makes 4 servings.

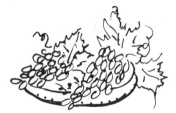

Aloha Mahi-Mahi

1 pound mahi-mahi
1 tablespoon lemon or lime juice
  salt
1/4 teaspoon marjoram
  barley flour
1 tablespoon milk-free margarine
1 tablespoon safflower oil
2 tablespoons milk-free margarine
1/4 cup sliced almonds, optional
2 tablespoons lemon or lime juice
1 lemon or lime, cut in wedges

Pompano, sole or turbot fillets can be used in this recipe. For an exciting garnish, try surrounding the fillets with a small papaya, halved, seeded, peeled and sliced and 1 avocado, peeled and sliced.

Season the fish with lemon juice, salt and marjoram. Dip in flour to coat and saute on both sides in margarine and oil. Fish will separate when fork-tested. Transfer to heated platter.

Add the 2 tablespoons of margarine to the pan along with the nuts and saute until golden brown. Add 2 tablespoons of lemon juice. Stir briskly, scraping up drippings and spoon over fish.

Garnish with lime or lemon wedges. Makes 4 servings.

Brook Trout Gourmet

4 brook trout
  seasoned barley flour
1/4 cup melted milk-free margarine
3 tablespoons milk-free margarine
  chopped watercress
  lemon wedges

Remove the fins, leaving the heads and tails on for a sophisticated touch.

Dip the brook trout into the seasoned flour.

Melt the 1/4 cup of milk-free margarine and saute the trout until they are firm and appear browned. Remove to a hot platter. Add the 3 tablespoons of milk-free margarine to the drippings in the pan and let the margarine brown slightly.

Sprinkle the fish with watercress, pour the browned margarine over the fish and garnish with the lemon wedges. Makes 4 servings.

Cod Francais

12 small, peeled potatoes
12 small white onions
   center cut of cod
   milk-free margarine
   dash thyme
1/4 teaspoon tarragon
1/4 teaspoon basil
   melted milk-free margarine

Garnish with chopped parsley or watercress and slices of lemon.

Parboil separately the potatoes and onions.

Place the cod in a shallow, ovenproof dish greased with milk-free margarine. Arrange onions and potatoes around the cod and then sprinkle with thyme, tarragon and basil.

Bake in a 350° oven for about 30 minutes, basting frequently with the melted margarine. Makes 4 servings.

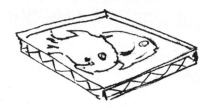

Bass Spectacular

1 1/4 cups orange juice
1/2 cup uncooked,
    long-grain white rice
3/4 cup pitted, diced dates
2 tablespoons milk-free margarine
2 tablespoons sugar
1/4 teaspoon ground ginger
1 whole sea bass (5 to 6 pounds),
    cleaned, scaled and left whole
1 large onion,
    peeled and thinly sliced
1/4 cup milk-free margarine, melted
3 oranges, peeled and sectioned

To serve with a flair, place the fish on a heated serving platter. Remove the skewers and spoon some stuffing onto the plate. Arrange the orange sections around the fish. For a taste surprise, sprinkle the oranges with a little cinnamon. A garnish of watercress will complete the picture.

In a medium saucepan, bring orange juice to a boil. Add rice and cover. Reduce heat and simmer until the rice is tender and the juice is absorbed, about 20 minutes. Add dates, milk-free margarine, sugar, and ginger. Stir to combine.

Carefully stuff the fish with the rice mixture and skewer closed. Arrange half of the onion rings in a 15x10-inch jelly roll pan and place the fish over the onions. Drizzle with the melted margarine, and then top with the remaining onion rings.

Bake in a 350° oven for 1 hour and 10 minutes or until the fish is tender and flakes easily with a fork. (If the fish is longer than the pan, aluminum foil under the head and tail will catch the drippings.) Makes 6 servings.

Cod con Lime Butter

1 pound cod fillets
1/4 cup barley flour
1/2 teaspoon paprika
1 1/2 teaspoons milk-free margarine
1 1/2 tablespoons safflower oil
  watercress or parsley sprigs
  lime slices

Also delicious with haddock fillets. Both can be fresh or frozen. If frozen, let thaw slightly at room temperature for 15 minutes.

Cut fillets crosswise into a total of 4 slices.

Combine flour and paprika and dredge the fillets.

Heat margarine and oil in a large skillet over medium-high heat. Cook the fish for about 5 minutes on each side. The fish will flake easily and be lightly browned when done. Transfer individual servings to separate plates. Spoon Lime Butter sauce over. Garnish with watercress and lime slices. Makes 4 servings.

SAUCE: In a small saucepan, melt 1/4 cup milk-free margarine over medium-low heat. Stir in 1 1/2 tablespoons lime juice and 3/4 teaspoon grated lime peel. Bring just to a boil with 1/8 teaspoon cilantro and 1/8 teaspoon basil. Spoon over each serving.

Salmon Saute

1 pound fresh salmon
2 tablespoons safflower oil
1 1/2 cups fresh broccoli flowerets
1 cup sliced, fresh mushrooms
1/2 cup green pepper,
  sliced lengthwise
1 clove garlic, minced
1/2 cup celery, sliced diagonally
2 tablespoons safflower oil
1/2 cup green onion,
  sliced diagonally
1/2 teaspoon grated lemon peel
1/4 teaspoon salt

Try sprinkling 2 tablespoons madeira over the salmon when adding the lemon peel and salt.

Skin and bone salmon and cut it into 1-inch cubes.

In a medium skillet, heat the 2 tablespoons of oil and saute the broccoli, mushrooms, green pepper, celery, and garlic over high heat until slightly tender. Remove the vegetables from the pan.

Add the second 2 tablespoons of oil to the skillet. Saute the salmon. Drain the excess oil.

Add the sauteed vegetables and the green onion. Sprinkle with the grated lemon peel and salt. Heat completely. Makes 2 to 3 servings.

Salmon Cups

1 can (15 1/2 oz.) salmon
1/2 cup finely chopped celery
1/4 cup finely chopped green pepper
2 tablespoons minced onion
1 tablespoon minced parsley
1 teaspoon egg substitute,
 plus 2 tablespoons water,
 beaten together
1/4 teaspoon lime juice
4 lemon slices

Drain and flake salmon.

Combine remaining ingredients except for lemon slices and mix together with salmon.

Place lemon slices on the bottom of 4 oiled (safflower oil) 6-ounce custard cups. Divide salmon mixture among the custard cups.

Place cups in a pan of boiling water and bake for 30 minutes at 350°. Makes 4 servings.

Baked Salmon

1 whole salmon,
   allow 1/2 pound per serving
   salt
   pepper
1 onion, peeled and chopped
1 green pepper, chopped
1 tablespoon milk-free margarine
1 tablespoon parsley

Clean the salmon, leaving the head and tail on. Salt and pepper the inside.

Combine the onion and green pepper and dot with the margarine. Stuff this onion mixture lightly into the fish.

Wrap the salmon in foil, sealing tightly and place carefully in a roasting pan. Bake in a 550° oven for 15 minutes. Lower the heat to 350° and finish baking at 10 minutes per pound. Serves according to the size of the fish at 1/2 pound per serving.

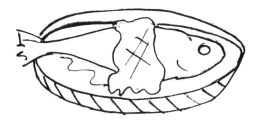

Scampi

1 1/2 pounds large raw shrimp
1/2 cup milk-free margarine
1/2 teaspoon salt
6 cloves garlic, peeled and crushed
3 tablespoons chopped parsley
1 teaspoon grated lemon peel
1 tablespoon lemon juice

Serve garnished with lemon wedges, or, for a sophisticated contrast with the lemon flavor, serve with lime wedges.

Preheat oven to 400º.

Shell shrimp, leaving the tails with shells. Devein and wash. Drain.

Melt margarine in a 9x13x2-inch baking dish in the oven. Add salt, garlic and 1 tablespoon of the parsley. Stir. Arrange shrimp in a single layer in the baking dish and bake, uncovered, 5 minutes.

Turn the shrimp; sprinkle with lemon peel, lemon juice, and remaining parsley. Bake 8 to 10 minutes longer or just until shrimp are tender.

Arrange shrimp on a heated serving platter and pour the garlic-margarine drippings over. Makes 4 servings.

Shrimp in Foil

8 medium shrimp,
  cleaned and deveined

1 tablespoon chopped scallions

8 thin slices water chestnuts

4 thin slices celery

12 thin carrot slices

1/4 teaspoon minced garlic

1/3 teaspoon salt

1 teaspoon milk-free margarine
  aluminum foil

Delicious for a quick luncheon or supper. Easy to prepare and even easier to clean up. The sauce is made while cooking and the shrimp can be served in the foil. Don't let that sauce go to waste. Pour it over rice and enjoy.

Arrange shrimp and remaining ingredients in the center of a 12-inch square of aluminum foil. Bring the corners of the foil together and pinch to make a tight bag. Place in a pot with 1 inch boiling water; cover tightly and cook 15 minutes or place on a shallow pan and bake 15 to 20 minutes in a 400° oven. Makes 1 serving.

Snow Crab Claws

2 packages (12 oz. each)
   Alaska Snow Crab claws
1 tablespoon milk-free margarine
2 cloves garlic, minced
1 tablespoon chopped green onion
1 tablespoon minced parsley
1/4 teaspoon cilantro
1/4 teaspoon chervil
1 tablespoon lemon juice
1/4 cup dry white wine

Thaw and drain crab claws.

Melt margarine with remaining ingredients. Add crab claws and simmer 3 minutes, basting frequently with sauce. Makes 6 servings.

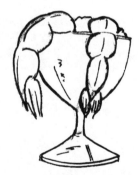

Vegetables

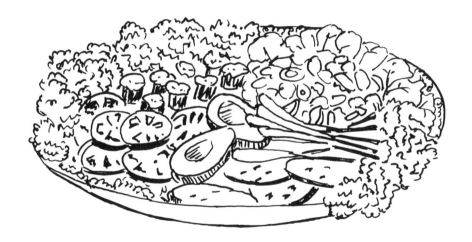

Broccoli and Asparagus Bouquet

2 tablespoons safflower oil
1 medium onion, thinly sliced
1 tablespoon shredded,
   fresh ginger root
1 clove garlic, crushed
1/2 teaspoon salt
3 cups fresh broccoli flowerets and
   stems, pared and sliced
   (about 3/4 pound)
1 pound fresh asparagus, trimmed and
   cut into 1-inch pieces
2 tablespoons freshly squeezed
   lemon juice
1 1/2 teaspoons sugar

Heat the oil in a large skillet. Cook the onions, ginger root, garlic and salt until the onions are soft, about 5 minutes.

Add broccoli and asparagus and stir to coat over high heat. Add lemon juice and sugar. Saute until vegetables are tender, 5 minutes or so. Makes 4 servings.

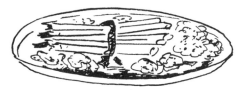

Herbed Broccoli

1 (10-oz.) package frozen,
   chopped broccoli
2 tablespoons milk-free margarine
1/4 cup sliced green onion
2 tablespoons diced pimiento
2 teaspoons lemon juice
1/2 teaspoon salt
1/4 teaspoon oregano
1/4 teaspoon chervil
1/4 teaspoon basil
1/8 teaspoon black pepper

Cook broccoli according to directions in a 2-quart saucepan and drain the water.

Add remaining ingredients; stir and serve. Makes 4 servings.

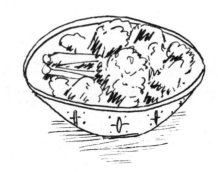

Gingered Carrots

7-8 medium carrots, cleaned
1/2 tablespoon brown sugar
1/2 tablespoon sugar
1 tablespoon arrowroot
1/4 teaspoon salt
1/4 teaspoon ginger
1/4 cup orange juice
2 tablespoons milk-free margarine
  parsley

Slice carrots crosswise, about 1/2-inch thick. Cook, covered, in salted water until just tender, about 20 minutes. Drain.

Combine sugars, arrowroot, salt, and ginger in another small saucepan. Add the orange juice and cook, stirring constantly until mixture becomes thick and bubbly. Boil 1 minute and stir in margarine.

Pour over hot carrots, tossing to coat evenly. Garnish with parsley. Makes 6 servings.

Carrot Pudding —Harriet Berner

1 1/2 cups barley flour
3 teaspoons cereal-free
  baking powder
1/2 teaspoon baking soda
1/2 teaspoon salt
1/2 teaspoon cinnamon
1/2 teaspoon nutmeg
1 teaspoon egg substitute,
  plus 2 tablespoons water
1 tablespoon water
2 cups grated carrots
1/4 cup safflower oil
1/2 cup packed brown sugar

Stir together all the ingredients up to and including the nutmeg.

Add the egg substitute along with the 2 tablespoons of water. Then add the 1 tablespoon water along with the carrots.

Add the oil and sugar.

Bake in a greased 1 1/2-quart mold or an 8x8-inch baking pan for 1 hour in a 350° oven. Cut into 9 to 12 pieces.

Braised Celery

1 1/2 pounds celery
3 tablespoons lemon juice
1/2 cup chicken stock
1/2 teaspoon salt
1 tablespoon sugar
2 tablespoons milk-free margarine
1/4 teaspoon chervil
1/4 teaspoon basil
1/4 teaspoon marjoram
1 tablespoon milk-free margarine

Wash and trim the celery. Arrange in a stovetop casserole dish.

Pour over the celery: lemon juice, stock, salt, sugar, and the first 2 tablespoons of margarine.

Bring the liquid to a boil. Place a lid over so that the steam escapes slightly and simmer for 25 minutes or until tender.

Remove the celery and keep warm. Continue heating liquid until there is about 1/2 cup left. Swirl in the 1 tablespoon margarine. Pour over the celery. Makes 4 servings.

VARIATIONS: Try Braised Belgian Endive or even Braised Boston Lettuce.

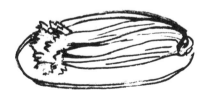

Butternut Squash

1 large butternut squash,
  pared, cut into 1-inch cubes,
  with seeds and fibers removed
1/4 teaspoon cinnamon
1/4 teaspoon nutmeg
1/2 cup packed brown sugar
2 teaspoons lime juice

Place squash cubes in 2-quart casserole or baking dish. Sprinkle with cinnamon, nutmeg, and sugar. Drizzle lime juice over.

Bake, uncovered, in a 375° oven for 45 minutes or until fork tender. Makes 4 servings.

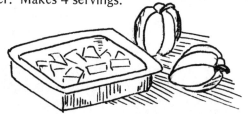

Tomatoes Herbed

2 large tomatoes
2 tablespoons milk-free margarine
1/4 cup crushed rice cereal or
  barley cereal
1/2 teaspoon salt
1/8 teaspoon oregano
1/8 teaspoon tarragon
1/4 teaspoon sugar

Wash tomatoes and cut in half. Place in shallow baking dish.

Melt margarine and combine with remaining ingredients. Spoon mixture evenly over tomatoes.

Bake in a 425° oven for 10 minutes. Makes 4 servings.

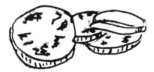

Barley Pilaf

3/4 cup milk-free margarine
1 pound mushrooms, sliced
4 medium onions, coarsley chopped
2 cups medium grain barley
4-5 cups chicken stock or broth
1 teaspoon salt
1/4 teaspoon pepper
1/4 teaspoon tarragon
1/4 teaspoon chervil

Melt margarine in a large skillet. Saute mushrooms and remove from pan.

Cook onions in margarine until soft, about 5 minutes. Add barley and cook until lightly browned, stirring frequently.

Add mushrooms and 2 cups of the stock to the barley. Season with salt, pepper, tarragon and chervil. Turn into a greased casserole.

Cover and bake at 350° for 30 minutes. Thus far, the recipe can be made ahead and frozen. On the serving day, add 1 cup of stock, cover and bake at 350° for 1 hour. Stir in the remaining cup of stock and bake 1 hour more. Uncover for the last 30 minutes. Makes 10 servings.

Saffron Rice

4 cups chicken stock
3/4 cup water
2 cups long grained rice
1/2 teaspoon powdered saffron
1/2 cup chopped onion
1/4 teaspoon basil
1/4 teaspoon chervil
2 tablespoons milk-free margarine
2 teaspoons salt

Bring chicken stock and water to a boil. Add remaining ingredients.

Stir and bring to a boil again. Reduce heat to simmer. Cover and cook until rice is tender, about 25 minutes. Makes 4 servings.

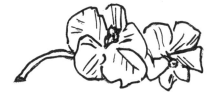

Rice Fritters

1 cup barley flour
3 teaspoons **cereal-free**
 baking powder
1/4 teaspoon salt
1 teaspoon egg substitute,
 plus 2 tablespoons water,
 beaten together
1 cup cooked rice
1/2 cup water
3 teaspoons chopped green onion
2 tablespoons milk-free margarine,
 melted

Stir together the flour, baking powder and salt.

Combine the beaten egg substitute and water, rice, 1/2 cup water, green onion and margarine.

Add the rice mixture to the dry ingredients, stirring until the flour is moistened.

Drop the batter by the rounded teaspoonful into deep safflower oil at 350°. Fry until golden brown, about 1 1/2 minutes per side, turning once. Drain on paper toweling and serve hot. Makes 32.

Mushroom, Potato Puff

3 medium baking potatoes,
  pared and cut up
  boiling water to cover
1/4 cup water
1 teaspoon egg substitute,
  plus 2 tablespoons water
1 tablespoon milk-free margarine
3/4 teaspoon salt
1/4 teaspoon **cereal-free**
  baking powder
1/2 cup chopped onion
4 tablespoons milk-free margarine
8 ounces fresh mushrooms, sliced
2 tablespoons snipped parsley

You can substitute coconut milk for the 1/4 cup of water.

Cook potatoes in boiling water until tender, 20 to 40 minutes and drain.

Place potatoes in bowl and beat until smooth. Add water, egg substitute and the 2 tablespoons water, salt and baking powder. Beat until fluffy.

Cook onion in margarine until tender. Add mushrooms and cook 3 minutes, until tender. Stir in parsley.

Line bottom and sides of a greased 8-inch pie plate with 1 1/2 cups of the potatoes, topping with the mushroom mixture. Spoon remaining potatoes evenly over, sealing the edges. Bake in a 400° oven for 15 to 18 minutes. Makes 6 servings.

Potato-Rutabaga Combo

1 pound rutabaga, cut in cubes
2 medium potatoes, cut in cubes
1/2 teaspoon salt
2 tablespoons milk-free margarine
1/2 cup chopped onion
2 tablespoons chopped parsley
1/2 teaspoon salt
1/8 teaspoon pepper

In a large saucepan, combine rutabagas and potatoes. Add water to cover and salt. Bring to a boil, then cover and reduce heat. Simmer for 30 to 40 minutes until the vegetables are tender.

While the vegetables are cooking, melt the margarine in a small saucepan. Add onion and parsley and cook until the onion is tender. Drain the vegetables and place them in a large bowl. Beat until smooth.

Stir in onions and parsley, salt and pepper, mixing well. Makes 4 to 6 servings.

Potato Pannicakes

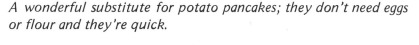

3 medium baking potatoes
2 tablespoons grated onion
2 tablespoons milk-free margarine
2 tablespoons safflower oil

A wonderful substitute for potato pancakes; they don't need eggs or flour and they're quick.

Wash and grate the potatoes on a medium grater along with the skin. Add the grated onion.

Melt the margarine and safflower oil in a skillet. Spread the potatoes about a quarter of an inch thick in the skillet and cook, covered, over medium low heat until browned on the bottom. Turn to brown the other side. Makes 4 servings.

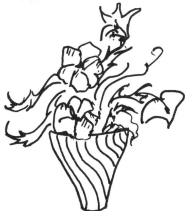

Oven Fried Potatoes

4 medium baking potatoes
1/4 cup melted milk-free margarine
  or safflower oil
1/2 teaspoon salt
1/4 teaspoon paprika

Preheat oven to 450º.

Pare the potatoes and cut them lengthwise into strips about 1/2 inch thick. Dry on paper towels. Spread in a single layer in a flat, ovenproof dish. Pour the melted margarine over the potatoes, turning the potatoes to coat well.

Bake about 30 to 40 minutes, turning 2 or 3 times. Drain on paper towels. Season with salt and paprika. Makes 4 servings.

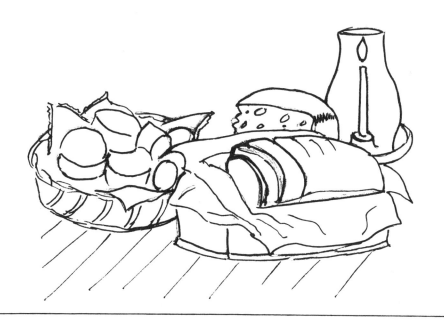

Individual Coffee Breads

1 cup sugar
1 cup applesauce
1/3 cup safflower oil
2 teaspoons egg substitute
   plus 4 tablespoons water
3 tablespoons water
2 cups barley flour
1 teaspoon baking soda
5 teaspoons cereal-free
   baking powder
1/2 teaspoon cinnamon
1/4 teaspoon salt
1/4 teaspoon nutmeg
3/4 cup chopped pecans, optional

You can also bake this recipe in a 9-cup, greased and floured, fluted cake pan in a 350º oven for 45 to 55 minutes, but the individual breads are elegant at a brunch or with morning coffee.

In a large bowl, thoroughly combine the sugar, applesauce, oil, egg substitute and water, and the 3 tablespoons water.

Stir together the flour and the remaining ingredients, but not the pecans. Add to the applesauce mixture and beat until well combined. Stir in the pecans if you are using them and then pour one half of the batter into 6 greased and floured (barley flour), 1-cup molds. Sprinkle filling over molds; pour remaining batter on top.

Bake in a 350º oven for 15 to 20 minutes. Cool 10 minutes in the molds and complete cooling on a wire rack. Makes 6 individual breads.

FILLING: Combine 1/4 cup brown sugar, 1/2 teaspoon cinnamon and 1/4 cup chopped pecans (optional).

Carrot Loaf

1 cup safflower oil
3/4 cup sugar
2 teaspoons egg substitute
  plus 4 tablespoons water
1 teaspoon vanilla
1 1/2 cups barley flour
1 1/2 teaspoons baking soda
1 1/2 teaspoons cinnamon
1/2 teaspoon salt
1 1/2 cups grated carrot

Stir together oil, sugar, egg substitute and water, and vanilla.

Stir together flour, baking soda, cinnamon and salt. Add to sugar mixture. Stir in carrots and mix just until blended.

Grease a 9x5-inch loaf pan and dust lightly with flour (barley flour). Bake in a 350° oven for 1 hour until center springs back if lightly pressed with finger. Cool cake in pan for 10 minutes and finish cooling on rack.

Raisin-Carrot Bread

2 1/2 cups barley flour
5 teaspoons cereal-free
  baking powder
1 1/2 teaspoons baking soda
1 teaspoon cinnamon
1 teaspoon salt
1 cup grated carrots
1 cup golden raisins
1/2 cup chopped walnuts, optional
1 cup well packed brown sugar
2 teaspoons egg substitute
  plus 4 tablespoons water
1 cup water
1/4 cup milk-free margarine, melted

Stir together flour, baking powder, baking soda, cinnamon and salt.

In a small bowl, combine carrots and raisins and toss. Blend in brown sugar.

In a large bowl, beat egg substitute and water together. Beat in the 1 cup of water and melted butter. Stir in carrot mixture and then add the flour mixture.

Bake in a greased 9-cup fluted tube pan in a 350° oven for 50 to 60 minutes. Cool in pan 5 to 10 minutes and finish cooling on a wire rack.

Applesauce Bread

1/2 cup milk-free margarine, softened
3/4 cup sugar
2 teaspoons egg substitute plus 4 tablespoons water
1 cup applesauce
1 teaspoon vanilla
1 teaspoon cinnamon
2 cups barley flour
1 teaspoon baking soda
1/2 teaspoon salt

In a large bowl, cream together the margarine and sugar.

Beat in the egg substitute and water and then the applesauce, vanilla and cinnamon.

Add the remaining ingredients, stirring by hand only until well blended.

Pour the batter into a 9x5-inch loaf pan, greased on the bottom only. Bake in a 350° oven for 50 to 60 minutes. Let cool ten minutes in the pan. Cool completely before slicing.

Honey of a Loaf

2 1/2 cups barley flour
6 1/4 teaspoons cereal-free
    baking powder
1/2 teaspoon baking soda
1 teaspoon salt
1 teaspoon egg substitute
    plus 4 tablespoons water
1 cup water
1 teaspoon vanilla
3/4 cup honey
2 tablespoons milk-free margarine,
    melted and cooled slightly
3/4 cup chopped dates, optional

Stir together the flour, baking powder, soda and salt.

Beat together the egg substitute and water along with the 1 cup of water, vanilla and honey.

Add melted margarine to the liquid mixture and beat the liquid mixture into the flour mixture until well blended.

Fold in the dates if you are using them.

Place the dough in a greased 9x5-inch loaf pan and bake in a 350° oven for 40 minutes. Cool 10 minutes in the pan and complete cooling on a wire rack.

Banana Bread

1/2 cup milk-free margarine,
  softened
1 cup sugar
2 teaspoons egg substitute
  plus 4 tablespoons water
1 cup ripe banana, mashed,
  (2 bananas)
1/4 cup water
1 teaspoon vanilla
2 cups barley flour
1 teaspoon soda
1/2 teaspoon salt

For an unusual flavor, add 1 tablespoon grated orange peel. This bread has a delicious, mild flavor.

In a large bowl, cream together the margarine and sugar.

Beat in the egg substitute and water and then the banana, water and vanilla.

Add the remaining ingredients, stirring by hand only until well combined.

Pour batter into a 9x5-inch loaf pan, greased on the bottom only. Bake in a 350° oven for 50 to 60 minutes. Let cool ten minutes in the pan. Cool completely before slicing.

VARIATION: HONEY BANANA BREAD: Use 1/2 cup of honey instead of sugar and 2 tablespoons water instead of 1/4 cup water.

Pumpkin Bread

1/2 cup milk-free margarine, softened
1 cup sugar
2 teaspoons egg substitute
  plus 4 tablespoons water
1 cup cooked pumpkin
1/4 cup water
1 teaspoon vanilla
1/2 teaspoon cinnamon
1/2 teaspoon nutmeg
1/4 teaspoon ginger
1 3/4 cups barley flour
1 teaspoon baking soda
1/2 teaspoon salt

For additional flavor and nutrition, add 1/2 cup raisins.

In a large bowl, cream together the margarine and sugar.

Beat in the egg substitute and water and then the pumpkin, water, vanilla and spices.

Add the remaining ingredients, stirring by hand only until well blended.

Pour batter into a 9x5-inch loaf pan, greased only on the bottom. Bake in a 350º oven for 50 to 60 minutes. Let cool ten minutes in the pan. Cool completely before slicing.

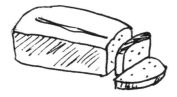

Date Bread

2 cups barley flour
1/3 cup sugar
5 teaspoons cereal-free
   baking powder
1 teaspoon salt
1 teaspoon egg substitute
   plus 2 tablespoons water
1 cup water
1/2 teaspoon vanilla
2 tablespoons milk-free margarine,
   melted and cooled slightly
3/4 cup chopped dates

For a richer flavor variation, substitute 1/2 cup brown sugar for the 1/3 cup of sugar.

Stir together the flour, sugar, baking powder and salt.

Beat the egg substitute and water along with the 1 cup of water and vanilla.

Add the melted margarine to the liquid mixture and beat the liquid mixture into the flour mixture until well blended.

Fold in the dates.

Pour the dough into a greased 9x5-inch bread pan and bake about 40 minutes in a 350° oven. Cool 10 minutes in the pan and complete cooling on a wire rack.

Lemon Bread

1 1/2 cups barley flour
1 cup sugar
3 3/4 teaspoons cereal-free
  baking powder
1/2 teaspoon salt
2 teaspoons egg substitute
  plus 4 tablespoons water
1/2 cup water
1/2 cup safflower oil
1 1/2 teaspoons grated lemon peel

For the finishing touch, use a wooden skewer to make holes in the loaf and then drizzle hot Lemon Glaze along the skewer into the holes.

In a large bowl, stir together the flour, sugar, baking powder and salt.

In a smaller bowl, beat egg substitute and water together with the 1/2 cup of water, oil, and lemon peel.

Add liquid mixture to flour mixture, mixing just until blended.

Pour batter into a greased and floured (barley flour) 9x5-inch loaf pan and bake in a 350° oven for 40 to 45 minutes. Let cool 5 minutes in pan. Finish cooling on a wire rack.

LEMON GLAZE: Heat 4 1/2 tablespoons lemon juice and 1/2 cup sugar until sugar dissolves.

Muffin Additions

1/2 cup chopped nuts or
1/2 cup chopped apricots or
1/2 cup chopped prunes or
1/2 cup chopped dates or
1/2 cup chopped figs or
1/2 cup mashed, ripe bananas or
1/2 cup chopped apples or
1/2 cup chopped cranberries plus
   2 teaspoons grated orange rind

In general, one adds the beaten liquid ingredients to the combined dry ingredients. Mixing should be minimal, not more than 20 seconds; ignore any lumps.

Spoon batter into greased muffin tins and fill each cup about two-thirds. If there is not enough batter to fill all the cups, put 4 tablespoons water in the empty cups.

Muffins are baked in a 400° oven for 20 to 25 minutes, unless individual recipes call for variable temperatures and times.

For variation, add the ingredients listed alongside to your muffins.

Cinnamon Dip Muffins

1/3 cup milk-free margarine
1/2 cup sugar
1 teaspoon egg substitute,
 plus 2 tablespoons water
1 1/2 cups barley flour
3 3/4 teaspoons cereal-free
 baking powder
1/2 teaspoon salt
1/2 cup water

Combine the margarine, sugar, and the egg substitute, along with the 2 tablespoons of water, beating until smooth.

Stir together the flour, baking powder and salt and add to the margarine mixture alternately with the water.

Spoon into 24 small, greased muffin cups, filling each 2/3 full and bake in a 400° oven for 15 to 18 minutes.

TOPPING: While the muffins are baking, melt 1/3 cup milk-free margarine. Combine 1 teaspoon cinnamon, 1/4 teaspoon nutmeg, and 1/2 cup sugar. When the muffins are baked, remove from the pans and dip them first into melted margarine and then into the sugar-spice mixture. Serve hot. Makes 24 small muffins.

Carrot Muffins

1 cup barley flour
1/4 cup packed brown sugar
2 1/2 teaspoons cereal-free
  baking powder
1/2 teaspoon salt
2 teaspoons egg substitute,
  plus 4 tablespoons water, beaten
1 cup carrots, finely shredded
1/4 cup safflower oil
1 tablespoon lemon juice

Thoroughly stir together the flour, sugar, baking powder and salt.

Combine egg substitute and water, carrots, safflower oil and lemon juice. Make a well in the dry ingredients and add to the dry ingredients all at once, stirring until just moistened.

Fill paper-lined muffin pans 2/3 full and bake in a 400° oven for 18 to 20 minutes. Makes 8 muffins.

Au Currant Muffins

3 tablespoons milk-free margarine
1/3 cup sugar
1 teaspoon grated orange peel
1 teaspoon egg substitute,
  plus 2 tablespoons water
1 1/2 cup barley flour
5 teaspoons cereal-free
  baking powder
1/2 teaspoon salt
1/2 teaspoon nutmeg
2/3 cup water
1/3 cup currants or raisins

Beat the margarine with the sugar until well blended and then beat in orange peel, egg substitute and the water for the egg substitute.

Stir together the flour, baking powder, salt and nutmeg.

Stir the flour mixture alternately with the water into the margarine-sugar mixture. Swirl in the currants.

Spoon into greased muffin cups, filling each about 2/3. Bake in a 375° oven for 20 to 25 minutes or until muffins are golden. Makes 12 muffins.

TOPPING: While muffins are baking, melt 1/2 cup milk-free margarine. Stir together 1 teaspoon cinnamon and 1/2 cup sugar. After muffins are baked, remove from pan and dip each muffin into the melted margarine and then into the cinnamon-sugar mixture.

Yam Muffins

1 3/4 cups barley flour
1/2 teaspoon salt
1/2 cup sugar
4 1/2 teaspoons cereal-free
   baking powder
1 teaspoon cinnamon
1/2 teaspoon nutmeg
2 teaspoons egg substitute,
   plus 4 tablespoons water
3 tablespoons milk-free margarine,
   melted
3/4 cup water
1 cup yams, cooked and mashed
2 teaspoons orange rind,
   grated, optional

Stir together the flour, salt, sugar, baking powder, and spices.

Beat the egg substitute and water and add the melted margarine, the water, and yams, and the grated orange rind.

Combine the liquid and the dry ingredients rapidly.

Fill well-greased muffin pans 2/3 full and bake in a 400° oven for 20 to 25 minutes. Makes 24 muffins.

Blueberry Muffins

2 ripe, medium bananas
2 teaspoons egg substitute,
  plus 4 tablespoons water
1 cup brown sugar, packed
1/2 cup milk-free margarine, melted
1/2 cup blueberries, washed
1 teaspoon vanilla
2 1/4 cups barley flour
5 1/2 teaspoons cereal-free
  baking powder
1/2 teaspoon cinnamon
1/4 teaspoon nutmeg
1/2 teaspoon salt

Slice bananas into a blender and puree.

Mix the pureed bananas with the egg substitute and water, the brown sugar, and melted margarine until well blended.

Stir in blueberrries and vanilla.

Stir together the flour, baking powder, cinnamon, nutmeg and salt. Make a well in the center of the flour and pour the liquid mixture in. Mix with a spoon just until blended. Spoon into well-greased 2 1/2-inch muffin cups. Bake in a 350° oven for 25 to 30 minutes. Makes 12 muffins.

Tangerine Muffins

2 cups barley flour
1/3 cup sugar
5 teaspoons cereal-free
 baking powder
1/2 teaspoon baking soda
1/2 teaspoon salt
1 cup rice cereal
2 teaspoons egg substitute,
 plus 4 tablespoons water,
 slightly beaten
1 cup tangerine juice
1/3 cup safflower oil

These muffins have variations galore. Try different cereals in place of rice cereal and try different juices—maybe an apricot nectar or a pear nectar.

Stir together the flour, sugar, baking powder and soda and salt. Stir in the cereal.

In a separate bowl, stir together the egg substitute, juice, and oil. Add all at once to the dry ingredients; mix only until just moistened.

Fill paper-lined muffin cups 2/3 full and bake in a 400° oven 20 to 25 minutes. Makes about 12 muffins.

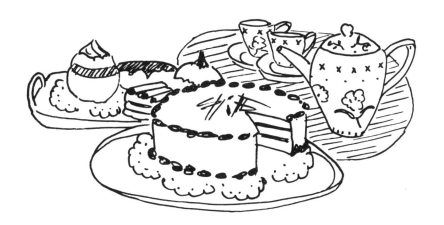

English Tea Ring

1/2 cup milk-free margarine
1 cup sugar
2 teaspoons egg substitute
  plus 4 tablespoons water
1/2 teaspoon almond extract
1/2 teaspoon vanilla
1 1/2 cups barley flour
3 3/4 teaspoons cereal-free
  baking powder
1/2 teaspoon salt
1/3 cup water
1/2 cup finely chopped
  pistachio nuts, optional
  confectioners' sugar, optional

Beat margarine and sugar until light and fluffy in a large bowl. Beat in egg substitute and water, 1 teaspoon of egg substitute and 2 tablespoons water at a time, beating well after each addition. Beat in almond extract and vanilla.

Stir together flour, baking powder and salt and add to margarine mixture a third at a time, alternately with the 1/3 cup water. Stir with a wire whip or beat at low speed until just blended. Fold in nuts, if used.

Pour into well-greased and floured (barley flour) 6-inch angel tube pan and bake in a 350° oven for 1 hour. Cool in pan for 5 minutes and turn out on rack to finish cooling. Wrap in aluminum foil or plastic wrap and store for a minimum of one day. Before serving, sift confectioners' sugar over the top.

Continental Tea Cake

1 cup milk-free margarine
1 1/4 cups sugar
2 1/4 cups barley flour
5 1/2 teaspoons cereal-free
  baking powder
1/2 teaspoon salt
1-2 tablespoons grated lemon peel
1/4 cup lemon juice
4 teaspoons egg substitute
  plus 8 tablespoons water

Cream the margarine. Gradually add sugar and continue beating until light and fluffy.

Add the remaining ingredients. Blend at low speed until moistened, then beat until blended, approximately 2 minutes.

Grease bottom only of a 9x13-inch pan. Pour batter in, spreading to edges. Bake in a 325° oven for 50-55 minutes. Cool completely.

Two-Layer Delight

3 cups barley flour
7 1/2 teaspoons cereal-free
  baking powder
1/2 teaspoon salt
1 cup milk-free margarine
1 1/2 cups sugar
2 teaspoons rum extract
1/2 teaspoon vanilla
4 teaspoons egg substitute
  plus 8 tablespoons water
6 tablespoons carob powder
  plus 4 tablespoons water
1 1/4 cups water

With rice flour, this cake has an excellent, delicious and subtle flavor. You may want to use less sugar since the carob is sweet. If you don't like the texture of the cake with the carob sauce, try baking the cake in a tube pan and eliminating the sauce.

Stir together flour, baking powder and salt.

Beat margarine in a large bowl, gradually adding sugar. Beat until fluffy. Beat in rum and vanilla and then beat in the egg substitute with water, 1 teaspoon of substitute and 2 tablespoons of water at a time. Slowly beat in the carob and water.

Add the flour mixture, one third at a time, alternately with water to the carob mixture, beating at low speed until just blended.

Grease two 9x9x2-inch pans. Line them with wax paper and then grease the wax paper. Pour the batter evenly into the two pans. Bake in a 350° oven for 35 to 40 minutes. Cool 10 minutes in pans. Loosen cake around the edges and turn out onto racks. Peel off the wax paper and cool the layers completely. *(continued)*

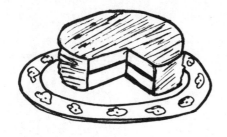

Carob Sauce to spread between the layers and drizzle on top.

In a small saucepan, combine 1 1/3 cups water, 2 teaspoons carob powder and 2 tablespoons brown sugar. Stir over a low flame and boil for one minute. Add 1 tablespoon butter and 1/2 teaspoon vanilla. Makes 1 cup.

Cafe Ole Cake

1/3 cup instant coffee
1/2 cup hot water
1 cup milk-free margarine
1 cup sugar
4 teaspoons egg substitute
  plus 8 tablespoons water
2 cups barley flour
5 teaspoons cereal-free
  baking powder
1/2 teaspoon salt

Coffee Glaze, page 178

For a milder flavor, use less instant coffee. For a finishing touch, top with Coffee Glaze or a sprinkle of confectioners' sugar.

Combine instant coffee and hot water.

Cream together margarine and sugar. Add egg substitute and water, one teaspoon of substitute and 2 tablespoons of water at a time, beating well after each addition.

Stir together the flour, baking powder and salt. Add alternately with coffee mixture to creamed margarine mixture.

Grease and flour (barley flour) a 9-cup fluted tube pan. Bake in a 350° oven for 40 to 50 minutes. Cool 10 minutes in the pan and turn out onto a wire rack to finish cooling.

Almond Torte

1 cup whole blanched almonds
1/3 cup barley flour
1 teaspoon cereal-free
  baking powder
3/4 cup sugar
1/4 cup milk-free margarine, melted
3 teaspoons egg substitute
  plus 6 tablespoons water
2 teaspoons vanilla extract
1/4 teaspoon almond extract
1 tablespoon grated lemon peel

Delicious, even without the glaze. For variation, try with peach, apricot or grape jam or any berry jam.

Line the bottom of a 9-inch round cake pan with wax paper and grease. Dust with flour (barley flour) and set aside.

Grind the almonds to a fine meal in an electric blender or a food processor. Add flour and baking powder; set aside.

In a mixing bowl, combine sugar, milk-free margarine, egg substitute and water, extracts and lemon peel and beat to blend well. Stir in the almond-flour mixture.

Bake in a 300° oven 35 to 40 minutes, until golden. Loosen edges and remove cake to serving plate. Makes 1 9-inch cake.

TOPPING: Combine 1/3 cup sugar and 1/4 cup lemon juice and brush over the hot cake. Cool. Slice and serve topped with a spoonful of raspberry preserves and a sprinkling of almonds.

Apricot Kuchen

1/2 cup milk-free margarine
3/4 cup sugar
2 teaspoons egg substitute
  plus 4 tablespoons water
1 teaspoon vanilla
1 cup barley flour
2 1/2 teaspoons creal-free
  baking powder
1/2 teaspoon salt
1 pound apricots, pitted, quartered

In a large bowl, beat together margarine and sugar until light and fluffy. Beat in egg substitute, one teaspoon substitute and 2 tablespoons water at a time. Add vanilla.

Stir together flour, baking powder and salt. Combine with margarine mixture and mix until well blended.

Spread batter evenly in lightly greased, 9x9-inch baking pan. Press apricots lightly on top of batter. Sprinkle with crumb topping. Bake in a 375° oven for 40 minutes. Top will be lightly browned. Cool in pan. Serve warm or cold.

TOPPING: Combine 1/2 cup sugar, 1/4 cup barley flour, 2 tablespoons milk-free margarine and 1/8 teaspoon cinnamon in a small bowl. Blend together with fingertips until crumbly.

Pear Cafe

2 1/4 cups barley flour
1 teaspoon baking soda
1/2 teaspoon salt
3/4 cup milk-free margarine
1 1/2 cups sugar
2 teaspoons egg substitute
  plus 4 tablespoons water
3/4 cup brewed, cold coffee
3 cups chopped, unpeeled fresh pears
  (2 large, 3-4 medium)

Stir together the flour, soda and salt.

Cream together milk-free margarine and sugar, beating in the egg substitute and water a teaspoon of substitute and 2 tablespoons of water at a time.

Stir in flour mixture alternately with coffee just until smooth and fold in the pears. Pour batter into a 13x9-inch baking pan that has been rubbed with milk-free margarine and sprinkle with topping. Bake in a 350º oven for 45 to 50 minutes. Serve warm. Makes 12 servings.

TOPPING: Combine 1 tablespooon cinnamon with 1/4 cup brown sugar and sprinkle over cake.

Honey Carrot Cake

1/2 cup milk-free margarine, softened
1/2 cup honey
2 teaspoons egg substitute
  plus 4 tablespoons water
1/2 teaspoon vanilla
2 medium carrots
1 cup barley flour
3/4 teaspoon baking soda
1/2 teaspoon salt
1/2 teaspoon cinnamon
1/2 teaspoon nutmeg

Cream together margarine, honey, egg substitute with water, and vanilla.

Shred carrots and add to the creamed mixture.

In another bowl, stir together remaining ingredients. Add carrot mixture to these ingredients and stir until blended.

Pour into an 8x8-inch pan, greased on the bottom only. Bake in a 375° oven for 25 to 30 minutes.

Brandied Gateau

3 cups coarsely chopped walnuts,
optional
1 1/2 cups maraschino cherries,
halved, optional because they
contain corn syrup
1 cup light raisins
1/2 cup dark raisins
3/4 cup barley flour
3/4 cup sugar
1 teaspoon cereal-free
baking powder
1/2 teaspoon salt
3 teaspoons egg substitute
plus 6 tablespoons water
2 tablespoons apricot brandy
or flavoring
1/2 cup apricot brandy
or flavoring

Combine nuts and fruits.

Stir together flour, sugar, baking powder and salt and add to fruit mixture. Toss to coat.

Beat egg substitute and water and add the 2 tablespoons brandy. Pour this brandy mixture over fruit mixture and mix well.

Pour into a greased and floured (barley flour) 9x5x3-inch loaf dish. Bake in a 300° oven for 1 hour, 45 minutes. Remove from oven and cool in pan.

Remove from pan. Moisten several layers of cheesecloth with 1/4 cup of the 1/2 cup of brandy. Wrap cake in cheesecloth and then wrap in foil. Store in the refrigerator. Two or three days later, moisten cheesecloth again with remaining brandy and wrap again in foil. Store in the refrigerator.

Banana Coffee Cake

1/2 cup milk-free margarine
3/4 cup sugar
1 3/4 cups barley flour
4 teaspoons cereal-free
  baking powder
1/2 teaspoon salt
1/2 teaspoon cinnamon
1/4 teaspoon baking soda
2 teaspoons egg substitute
  plus 4 tablespoons water,
  beaten together
2 ripe, medium bananas,
  mashed (1 cup)
1/4 cup water
1 teaspoon vanilla

Cream margarine and sugar and add 3/4 cup of the flour. Stir until mixture resembles coarse crumbs. Set aside 1/2 cup of this sugar-flour mixture for the topping.

Stir the remaining 1 cup of flour together with baking powder, salt, cinnamon, baking soda, egg substitute and water, bananas and 1/4 cup water.

Add the banana mixture to the sugar-flour mixture not reserved for topping, stirring until just mixed.

Turn into a greased 9x9x2-inch baking pan and sprinkle with the mixture reserved for the topping. Bake in a 375° oven for 25 to 30 minutes.

Cherry Coffee Cake

1 1/4 cups barley flour
1/2 cup sugar
3 1/4 teaspoons baking powder
1/4 teaspoon salt
1/4 cup milk-free margarine
1 teaspoon egg substitute
  plus 2 tablespoons water,
  beaten together
3 tablespoons water
1 teaspoon vanilla
3 cups fresh, pitted cherries
1 cup sugar
3 tablespoons barley flour
1/4 teaspoon almond extract
  or, if using canned, pitted, tart
  red cherries,
(continued)

Delicious with fresh or canned cherries. Try it both ways.

In a mixing bowl, stir together the flour, sugar, baking powder and salt. Cut in margarine until the mixture looks like coarse crumbs.

Combine the beaten egg substitute and water, the 3 tablespoons water, and vanilla and add to the dry ingredients, stirring well.

Spread into a greased 11x7½x1½-inch baking pan. If you are using fresh cherries, combine the cherries, sugar, barley flour and almond extract. Spoon cherry mixture over the top of the cake and sprinkle with topping. If you are using canned cherries, combine cherries, juice, almond extract, sugar and tapioca and let stand for 20 minutes before spooning mixture over cake. Sprinkle with topping. Bake in a 350° oven for 45 to 50 minutes. Serves 12.

TOPPING: Combine 1/2 cup barley flour, 1/4 cup brown sugar and 1/2 teaspoon cinnamon. Cut in 1/4 cup milk-free margarine until mixture resembles coarse crumbs.

3 cups canned cherries
3/4 cup juice from canned cherries
1/4 teaspoon almond extract
1 cup sugar
2 tablespoons quick cooking tapioca

Cinnamon Swirls

1 3/4 cups barley flour
4 1/2 teaspoons cereal-free
  baking powder
1/4 teaspoon salt
1/2 teaspoon cinnamon
1 cup milk-free margarine
1 cup sugar
4 teaspoons egg substitute
  plus 8 tablespoons water
1 teaspoon vanilla

Stir together the flour, baking powder, salt and cinnamon.

In a second bowl, cream margarine and then gradually add sugar while beating. Beat until light and fluffy. Beat in the egg substitute and water, 1 teaspoon of egg substitute and 2 tablespoons of water at a time.

Add half of the flour mixture to the butter mixture and blend. Then blend in the remaining flour mixture and vanilla *just* until ingredients are moistened.

Grease and flour (barley flour) a one-cup muffin mold and pour batter in. Do not fill each cup completely. Bake in a 325° oven for 25 to 30 minutes. Cool 10 minutes in pan before removing. Makes 6 mini coffee cakes.

Seed Cake

3/4 cup milk-free margarine
2 cups sugar
4 teaspoons egg substitute
  plus 8 tablespoons water
4 teaspoons grated lemon peel
3 cups barley flour
7 1/2 teaspoons cereal-free
  baking powder
1/2 teaspoon nutmeg
1 cup water
1 tablespoon caraway seed
1 tablespoon poppy seed
1 tablespoon anise seed

Cream margarine and sugar together until fluffy. Mix in egg substitute and water, one teaspoon of egg substitute and 2 tablespoons water at a time, blending thoroughly. Add lemon peel.

Stir together flour, baking powder and nutmeg. Add to butter mixture alternately with the 1 cup of water and blend well.

Spread with margarine and flour (barley flour) a 10-inch tube pan or a 12-cup fluted tube pan. Spoon one half of the batter into the pan and sprinkle caraway seeds on top. Cover with one third of the remaining batter and sprinkle with poppy seeds. Top with one half of the remaining batter and sprinkle with anise seeds. Spoon in rest of batter and bake in a 350° oven for 1 hour. Let cool in pan for 10 to 15 minutes and turn out onto a wire rack to continue cooling.

Applesauce Coffee Cake

1/2 cup milk-free margarine, softened
1/2 cup sugar
3/4 cup barley flour
2 teaspoons egg substitute
   plus 4 tablespoons water,
   beaten together
1 teaspoon vanilla
1 cup barley flour
4 1/2 teaspoons cereal-free
   baking powder
1/2 teaspoon baking soda
1/2 teaspoon salt
1 cup chunk-style applesauce
1/4 cup chopped nuts, optional
1 teaspoon cinnamon

For a sweeter coffee cake, add 1/4 cup more sugar. For the more crumbly texture of a coffee cake, cream the margarine and sugar together with a fork and stir in the 3/4 cup of flour with a fork.

Cream together the margarine and sugar. Add the 3/4 cup of flour and stir until crumbly. Set aside 1/2 cup.

To the remaining crumb mixture, add egg substitute and water and vanilla and, using a mixer, beat until smooth.

Stir together the 1 cup of barley flour, baking powder, soda and salt. Add alternately with applesauce to creamed mixture, beating after each addition.

Turn into a greased 10-inch pie plate. Stir nuts and cinnamon into reserved 1/2 cup crumb mixture and sprinkle over batter. Bake in a 375° oven 30 to 35 minutes.

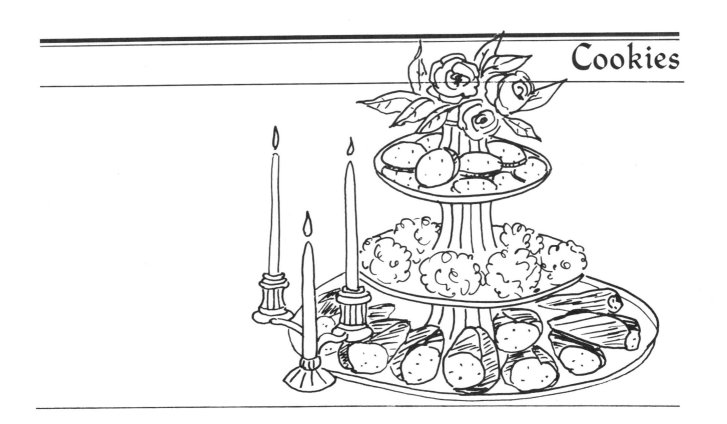

Cookies

Pumpkin Cookies

1/2 cup milk-free margarine, softened
1/4 cup sugar
1/4 cup brown sugar
1 teaspoon egg substitute
  plus 2 tablespoons water
1/2 cup cooked pumpkin
1 teaspoon vanilla
1 cup barley flour
1 1/4 teaspoons
  cereal-free baking powder
1/4 teaspoon salt
1 teaspoon cinnamon
1/4 teaspoon nutmeg
1/8 teaspoon ginger
1/2 cup raisins, optional

Cream margarine and sugars. Beat in egg substitute and water, pumpkin and vanilla. Stir in remaining ingredients until well blended.

Drop by the teaspoonful 1 inch apart onto a lightly greased baking sheet. Bake in a 350° oven for 15 to 18 minutes or until center is set. Makes 48 cookies.

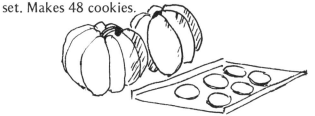

Pumpkin Treats

1/4 cup milk-free margarine
1/2 cup sugar
1/2 cup brown sugar, packed
1 can (1/2 pound) cooked pumpkin
1 teaspoon vanilla
2 teaspoons egg substitute
   plus 4 tablespoons water
3/4 cup barley flour
2 teaspoons baking powder
1/4 teaspoon baking soda
1/8 teaspoon salt
1 1/4 teaspoons pumpkin pie spice
1/2 cup raisins

Melt milk-free margarine. Stir in sugars, pumpkin, vanilla and the 2 teaspoons egg substitute plus 4 tablespoons water. Beat well. Stir in remaining ingredients until well mixed.

Pour into greased 9x13-inch pan and bake in a 350° oven for 20 to 25 minutes until top springs back when lightly touched. Cool. Makes 37 to 40 bars.

Pepparkahar

1 cup milk-free margarine, softened
1 1/2 cups sugar
3 tablespoons molasses
1 teaspoon egg substitute
   plus 2 tablespoons water
2 tablespoons water
3/4 cup barley flour
2 tablespoons baking soda
1/2 teaspoon salt
2 teaspoons cinnamon
1 1/2 teaspoons ginger
1 teaspoon cloves
1/2 teaspoon cardamom, optional

You may find that a little sugar sprinkled on the floured board, on the dough, and on the cookie cutter makes the dough easier to handle.

Cream together margarine, sugar and molasses. Beat in the egg substitute plus 2 tablespoons water along with 2 tablespoons water. Stir in remaining ingredients until combined.

Roll out on barley floured surface to 1/8-inch thickness. Cut with barley floured cookie cutter. Place 1 inch apart on ungreased baking sheet. Bake in a 350° oven for 7 to 10 minutes. Remove to cool on wire rack. Makes 30 cookies.

Shortbread Squares

1 1/4 cups barley flour
1/4 cup sugar
1/2 cup milk-free margarine
1 1/3 cups flaked coconut
2/3 cup pure maple syrup
1/4 teaspoon salt

Stir together the flour and sugar. Cut in margarine until mixture resembles fine crumbs.

Press mixture into 8x8x2-inch baking pan. Bake in a 375° oven for 15 to 20 minutes.

Combine coconut, syrup and salt in a small saucepan. Cook, stirring often, until coconut absorbs most of syrup, about 8 to 10 minutes. Spread over warm crumb mixture and return to oven for 10 minutes. While warm, cut into small bars. Makes 24 bars.

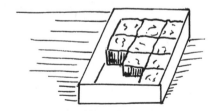

Woven Crowns

2 1/2 cups barley flour
1 cup milk-free margarine
1/2 cup sugar
3 tablespoons apricot brandy, optional
2 teaspoons vanilla
1 teaspoon water

When working the dough, add a few drops of water for a soft dough if necessary.

Combine all the ingredients.

Work with your hands to form a soft dough. You may color half of the dough if you wish.

Using a rounded teaspoonful of dough, roll on a lightly floured (barley flour) surface with hands to form 5-inch ropes. Twist 2 ropes together. Place on a greased cookie sheet and bake in a 350° oven for 13 to 15 minutes. Makes 18 or more cookies, depending upon the size of the ropes.

Lemon Balls

1/2 cup milk-free margarine
2/3 cup sugar
2 teaspoons grated lemon peel
1 teaspoon egg substitute
  plus 2 tablespoons water
1 3/4 cups barley flour
1/2 teaspoon salt
1/4 teaspoon baking soda
1/4 teaspoon cream of tartar
3 tablespoons lemon juice
1 tablespoon water
  confectioners' sugar

Beat together the milk-free margarine, sugar and lemon peel until creamy. Beat in egg substitute and water until fluffy.

Combine flour with salt, baking soda and cream of tartar. Add the flour mixture to the creamed mixture alternately with the combined lemon juice and water. Mix until just blended.

With floured hands, form the dough into 1-inch balls. Place about 1 inch apart on ungreased baking sheets. Bake in a 350° oven for 15 to 18 minutes until very light brown and firm to touch. Cool on wire racks. Gently shake a few at a time in a small bag of confectioners' sugar. Cool completely. Makes 42 cookies.

Rum Balls

2 cups barley flour
2 teaspoons ground nutmeg
1/2 teaspoon salt
1 cup milk-free margarine
3/4 cup sugar
2 teaspoons vanilla
2 teaspoons rum flavoring
1 teaspoon egg substitute
   plus 2 tablespoons water

Store these cookies up to three days with waxed paper between layers in covered containers. You can also freeze them.

Combine flour, nutmeg, and salt.

Beat together the margarine and sugar until creamy. Beat in the vanilla, rum flavoring, egg substitute and water until fluffy.

Stir flour mixture into the creamed mixture until blended.

Cover bowl and chill for at least 2 hours. With floured hands, form dough into 1-inch balls. (If crumbly, let dough stand at room temprature about 15 minutes.)

Place balls on ungreased baking sheet about 1 inch apart. Bake in a 350⁰ oven for 12 to 15 minutes until lightly browned. Remove from sheets and cool on wire racks. Makes 48 cookies.

FROSTING: Beat together 1/4 cup milk-free margarine, 1 teaspoon rum flavoring, 1/2 teaspoon vanilla and 2 1/2 cups unsifted confectioners' sugar. Add 2 to 3 tablespoons water for spreading consistency. Frost after icing sets up.

155

Crosshatch Cookies

1 cup milk-free margarine
1/2 cup unsifted confectioners' sugar
1/2 teaspoon vanilla
1/2 teaspoon almond extract
2 cups flour
1/4 teaspoon salt
1 cup finely chopped almonds,
  optional

These cookies may be stored at room temperature for up to 3 days when covered tightly or frozen with waxed paper between layers.

Beat the margarine until creamy. Beat in sugar, vanilla and almond extract until fluffy. Blend in flour, salt and 1/2 cup of the almonds until smooth.

With floured hands, form dough into 1-inch balls. Roll balls in remaining 1/2 cup almonds to coat, then place about 1 1/2 inches apart on slightly greased baking sheet. Flatten with the tines of a fork dipped into barley flour in a crisscross pattern. Bake until lightly browned in a 325° oven for 20 to 25 minutes. Remove cookies from sheet and cool on wire racks. Makes 48 cookies.

Lemony Crinkles

3/4 cup milk-free margarine
3/4 cup sugar
1 teaspoon egg substitute
  plus 2 tablespoons water
1/2 teaspoon vanilla
1/2 teaspoon lemon extract
1/4 cup water
2 cups barley flour
5 teaspoons
  cereal-free baking powder
1/2 teaspoon salt
1/4 teaspoon baking soda
1/2 cup sugar
1 tablespoon grated lemon rind

Beat margarine with sugar until fluffy. Beat in egg substitute with water, vanilla, lemon extract and the 1/4 cup of water.

Stir together flour, baking powder, salt and baking soda. Add to margarine mixture a little at a time, blending after each addition.

Chill dough several hours or until firm. Using a teaspoonful of dough, form it into a ball by rolling lightly between your palms.

Coat the balls by rolling in a mixture of sugar and lemon rind. Place 2 inches apart on cookie sheets. Bake in a 350° oven for 10 to 12 minutes until cookie edges are lightly browned. Cool on a wire rack. Makes 60 cookies.

Carob Cookies

1 1/2 cups barley flour
1 teaspoon cream of tartar
1/2 teaspoon baking soda
1/4 teaspoon salt
1/2 cup milk-free margarine
1 teaspoon egg substitute
   plus 2 tablespoons water
1/2 cup sugar
1 teaspoon vanilla
1 ounce carob chips, melted

Stir together the flour, cream of tartar, baking soda and salt. With a pastry blender, cut in the milk-free margarine until fine.

Beat the egg substitute and water with sugar and vanilla and stir into the flour mixture. Stir in the melted carob until blended and smooth.

Roll level teaspoonsful of the dough into balls. Place several inches apart on greased cookie sheets; they will spread. With the palm of your hand, flatten each cookie to about ¼-inch thickness.

Bake in a 375º oven for 8 to 10 minutes. Let cool 1 or 2 minutes on the sheet before removing to a wire rack to finish cooling. Makes about 24 cookies.

Brown Sugar Cookies

1/2 cup milk-free margarine
1/3 cup sugar
1/3 cup brown sugar, packed
1 teaspoon egg substitute
    plus 2 tablespoons water
1 tablespoon water
1/2 teaspoon vanilla
1 1/4 cups barley flour
1/2 teaspoon baking soda
1/4 teaspoon salt
1/2 cup carob chips

Cream together the milk-free margarine and sugars. Add egg substitute with water, the 1 tablespoon of water and vanilla; beat well.

Stir together the flour, soda and salt and blend into the creamed mixture. Stir in the chips by hand.

Drop the cookies from a teaspoon about two inches apart on a greased cookie sheet and bake in a 350º oven for 12 to 14 minutes. Makes 42 cookies.

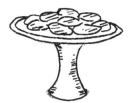

Carob Sandies

3/4 cup milk-free margarine
1/3 cup sugar
3 tablespoons water
1 teaspoon vanilla
1 3/4 cups barley flour
1/2 cup carob chips
   sifted confectioners' sugar

Cream together the milk-free margarine and sugar until light and fluffy. Beat in water and vanilla and blend in flour. Stir in carob chips.

Shape dough into balls, using about 2 tablespoons dough for each.

Place balls on ungreased cookie sheet and bake in a 325° oven for 20 minutes. Remove to cooling rack. While cookies are warm, sprinkle them with confectioners' sugar. Makes 54 cookies.

Carob Crinkles

1 cup milk-free margarine
1 3/4 cups sifted confectioners' sugar
2 tablespoons water
1 teaspoon vanilla
8 ounces carob chips or bars, grated
  (run through the blender)
2 cups barley flour
  dash of salt

Cream together the milk-free margarine and confectioners' sugar. Beat in vanilla along with 2 tablespoons of water. Add the carob and flour along with a dash of salt and blend well.

Shape into 1-inch balls and place on an ungreased cookie sheet.

Bake in a 325° oven for 25 minutes and sprinkle with confectioners' sugar if desired. Makes 72 cookies.

Frosted Bars

6 tablespoons milk-free margarine, softened

3/4 cup sugar

1 teaspoon egg substitute plus 2 tablespoons water

2 tablespoons water

3/4 teaspoon vanilla

1 1/2 cups barley flour

1/2 teaspoon baking soda

1/2 teaspoon salt

Cream together the milk-free margarine and sugar. Beat in egg substitute and water along with the 2 tablespoons of water and the vanilla.

Stir together the flour with baking soda and salt. Add the flour mixture to the creamed mixture and blend well.

Pour into a greased 9x9-inch baking pan and bake in a 375° oven for 20 to 25 minutes. Makes 12 bar cookies.

FROSTING: In a saucepan, combine 1/3 cup packed brown sugar, 2 tablespoons milk-free margarine and 2 tablespoons water. Bring to a boil, stirring constantly. Remove from heat and stir in 1 teaspoon vanilla. Gradually stir in 1 cup sifted powdered sugar. If the mixture is too thick, add a few drops of hot water until the frosting is of spreading consistency. Spread over warm cookies immediately and cut into bars.

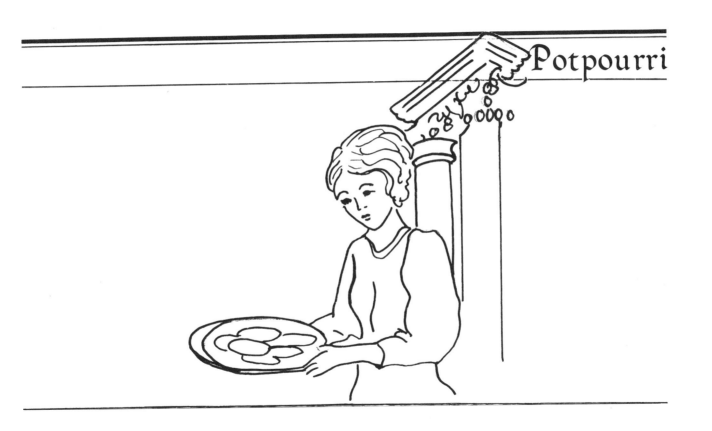

Potpourri

Pancakes

1 1/4 cups barley flour
3 1/8 teaspoons cereal-free
   baking powder
1 tablespoon sugar
1/4 teaspoon salt
1 teaspoon egg substitute
   plus 2 tablespoons water, beaten
1 cup water
2 tablespoons safflower oil

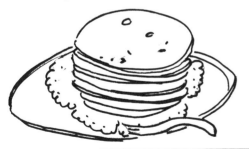

Stir together the dry ingredients.

Combine the egg substitute and water along with the cup of water and oil and add to dry ingredients. Stir just until moistened. Batter will be lumpy.

Using a quarter-cup measure, (or a tablespoon for dollar pancakes), bake on a hot griddle. (Water drops dance when the griddle is hot enough.) Turn when the unbaked tops are bubbly. Makes 8 4-inch pancakes or 12 dollar pancakes.

VARIATIONS:

BLUEBERRY PANCAKES: Add 1 cup blueberries to batter.
APPLE PANCAKES: Add 2 apples, shredded and 1/2 teaspoon cinnamon to batter.
BANANA PANCAKES: Press slices of banana on each pancake as it bakes on griddle.
HAM PANCAKES: Add 1/4 cup cubed ham to batter.
NUT PANCAKES: Add 1/4 cup chopped nuts to batter.

Pumpkin Waffles

2 1/4 cups barley flour
6 teaspoons cereal-free
   baking powder
2 teaspoons cinnamon
1 teaspoon ginger
1/4 teaspoon nutmeg
1/2 teaspoon salt
1/4 cup brown sugar
1 cup canned pumpkin
2 cups water
1/4 cup melted milk-free margarine
4 teaspoons egg substitute,
   plus 8 tablespoons water

These waffles are far superior to any we have tested. They are crisp, have good color and are delicious. You can even freeze them and pop them into the toaster.

Stir together the flour, baking powder, spices, salt and sugar.

Combine the pumpkin and water. Add the flour mixture and the melted margarine. Stir to blend.

Beat the egg substitute and water until bubbly and fold into batter to blend.

When waffle iron is ready, pour batter onto grill and cook until waffles are richly browned and crisp, about 5 minutes. Makes about 12 waffles.

Breakfast Muffins

4 cups rice cereal
1 cup barley flour
2 1/2 teaspoons
  cereal-free baking powder
1/4 teaspoon salt
2 teaspoons egg substitute
  plus 4 tablespoons water
1 cup water
1/4 cup milk-free margarine, melted
1/4 cup raisins, optional

Crush rice cereal; 4 cups should come to 1 cup of crumbs.

Combine remaining ingredients until just blended.

Pour into paper muffin cups and bake in a 400° oven for 20 minutes. Makes 12 to 16 muffins.

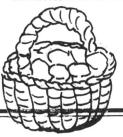

Breakfast Bananas

Peel and cut firm bananas in half, lengthwise. Sandwich pineapple spears in between the banana halves and wrap with bacon slices. Broil in a pan, turning frequently until the bacon is crisp.

Breakfast Bacon Muffins

1/2 cup milk-free margarine
1 cup sugar
2 teaspoon egg substitute,
  plus 4 tablespoons water
1 cup banana, mashed
1/2 cup yam, mashed
  1 (8-oz. can) or
  1 small yam, baked and mashed
6 slices of bacon,
  cooked and crumbled
1 1/2 cups barley flour
3 3/4 teaspoons cereal-free
  baking powder
1/2 teaspoon cinnamon
1/4 teaspoon salt
1/8 teaspoon nutmeg
1/3 cup water

Cream together the margarine and sugar until light and fluffy.

Beat in the egg substitute and water and add the banana and yam along with the crumbled bacon. Blend well.

Stir together the flour, baking powder, cinnamon, salt and nutmeg.

Stir the flour mixture into the creamed margarine mixture alternately with water and then spoon into 16 greased 2 1/2-inch muffin pan cups. Bake in a 400° oven for 20 to 25 minutes. Makes 16 muffins.

VARIATIONS: MUFFIN POULET: Substitute 1 cup of cooked chicken meat either shredded or chunked for the bacon.
MUFFIN BOEUF: Substitute 1 cup of cooked beef either shredded or chunked for the bacon.

Favorite Stuffing

2 small onions, peeled and minced
2 stalks celery,
   thinly sliced crosswise
1 tablespoon milk-free margarine
2 carrots, peeled and
   coarsely shredded
2 yams, peeled and
   coarsely shredded
1/2 cup parsley tops

Our thanks to Esther Tenenbaum for this unusual stuffing. It's not only excellent inside the turky, try baking it separately in a 350⁰ oven. It is delicious as a side dish and there's always enough to go around.

Simmer the onions and celery in margarine until golden.

Combine the onions and celery with the remaining ingredients and spoon into turkey. Stuffs a 9 pound turkey.

Water Chestnut Stuffing

1 cup cooked rice,
  wild rice or precooked rice, using
  chicken stock instead of water
1 heaping tablespoon raisins
1 (8-oz.) can water chestnuts,
  sliced thin
3 tablespoons fresh parsley,
  chopped
  chicken liver, minced
2 tablespoons milk-free margarine,
  softened

Combine ingredients and stuff bird. Makes sufficient stuffing for a 3 1/2 to 4-pound bird.

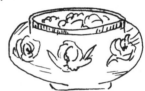

Apple Raisin Dressing

6 cups puffed rice
1 medium onion, finely chopped
1 1/2 cups celery, finely chopped
2 cups tart apples, chopped
  (about 2 large apples)
1/2 cup raisins
2 tablespoons lemon juice
1/8 tablespoon tarragon
2 tablespoons milk-free margarine,
  melted

Combine all ingredients up to and including the raisins.

Sprinkle lemon juice, tarragon and melted margarine over rice mixture. Toss thoroughly and stuff bird. Makes about 6 cups of dressing. Recipe can be doubled for larger bird.

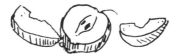

Wild Rice Dressing

giblets
4 cups water
1 teaspoon salt
1 cup wild rice
1/4 cup milk-free margarine
2 tablespoons shallots, chopped
1/4 cup chopped celery
1/4 cup jicama, pared and sliced
1 cup mushrooms, sauteed

Chop the giblets. Bring the water and salt to a boil and simmer the giblets for 15 minutes. Remove the giblets and bring the water to a strong boil. Stir in the wild rice and simmer about 30 minutes.

Melt the margarine in a skillet and saute the shallots, celery and jicama.

Add the hot, drained rice, chopped giblets, and mushrooms. Makes about 3 cups.

Apple Dressing

6 cups tart cooking apples
1 cup raisins
2 tablespoons lemon juice

Pare and slice the apples and combine them with the raisins and lemon juice. Makes 4 cups.

Marinades for Pork Roast

WINE MARINADE

1 cup dry wine
2 cloves garlic, sliced
2 teaspoons salt
1/4 teaspoon pepper
2 tablespoons minced parsley
1/2 teaspoon chervil
1/2 teaspoon basil

Combine all ingredients. Marinate a pork roast for 2 to 4 hours at room temperature or overnight in refrigerator.

HERB MARINADE

1/2 cup dry white wine
1/2 cup safflower oil
1/4 cup vinegar
   (avoid if mold sensitive)
1 teaspoon salt
1 teaspoon oregano
1 teaspoon basil
1/2 teaspoon marjoram
1/2 teaspoon cilantro
2 cloves garlic, minced

Combine all ingredients. Marinate a pork roast for 2 to 4 hours at room temperature or overnight in refrigerator.

Raisin Sauce

1/2 cup packed brown sugar
2 tablespoons arrowroot
1 teaspoon dry mustard
1 tablespoon vinegar
  (avoid if mold sensitive)
1 cup raisins
1/4 teaspoon grated lemon peel
2 tablespoons lemon juice

Try this sauce with ham.

Combine the first 3 ingredients in a saucepan. Slowly add the vinegar and then the remaining ingredients along with 1 1/2 cups of water. Stir over medium heat until thick and bubbly. Serve hot. Makes 2 1/2 cups.

Cranberry Sauce

Wash 1 pound of cranberries. Put them in a saucepan and cover with 2 cups of boiling water. When the water returns to a boil, cover and continue boiling for 3 to 4 minutes. When the skins burst, put them through a strainer or ricer and stir in 2 cups sugar. Bring to a boil and remove from the heat.

Glazes for Ham

1 cup packed brown sugar
2 tablespoons barley flour
1/2 teaspoon dry mustard
1/8 teaspoon cinnamon
3 tablespoons dry sherry
   or water

BROWN SUGAR

Mix well and spread on ham before baking.

1 cup orange marmalade

MARMALADE

Spread marmalade on ham before baking.

1 cup packed brown sugar
3/4 cup drained, crushed pineapple

PINEAPPLE

Combine sugar and pineapple. Spread on ham before baking.

Caramel Topping

1/4 cup milk-free margarine
1 cup brown sugar, packed
2 tablespoons honey
1 teaspoon cinnamon
1/2 teaspoon chopped lemon rind,
  optional

This topping is put on the bottom of a roll pan and when the rolls are popped out, it becomes the topping.

Melt the margarine in a saucepan and then stir in the sugar, honey, cinnamon and lemon rind. Makes enough for 12 rolls.

Honey Glaze

1/2 cup sugar
1/4 cup water or coconut milk
1/4 cup milk-free margarine
1/4 cup honey

In a saucepan, stir together the sugar, water, margarine and honey while bringing to a boil. Glazes a 9x13-inch coffee cake that is ready for baking.

Streusel

2 tablespoons rice flour
2 tablespoons milk-free margarine
5 tablespoons sugar
1/2 teaspoon cinnamon

Use this topping before baking.

Combine the flour, margarine and sugar with a fork until they are crumbly in texture.

Add cinnamon and stir to blend.

Sprinkle over the cake. Makes enough for an 8x8-inch cake.

Coffee Glaze

1/4 cup strong, hot coffee
1/4 cup sugar
1/2 teaspoon cinnamon

Into the coffee, stir the sugar and cinnamon.

Just before the end of the baking time, brush on the coffee glaze.

VARIATIONS: Instead of coffee, dissolve the sugar and cinnamon in hot water. Also, try brown sugar instead of white.

Honey Glaze II

2 tablespoons sugar
1/4 cup honey
1 tablespoon milk-free margarine

This honey glaze is applied to cakes that have already been baked.

Combine the ingredients and bring to a boil.

Pie Crust I

1 1/3 cups barley flour
1 teaspoon salt
1 stick milk-free margarine
1/4 cup ice water

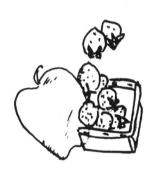

This dough may be easier to make using a food processor. If you have difficulty rolling this dough out, simply pat it on the bottom and sides of an 8-inch pie plate.

Blend the first three ingredients.

While continuing to blend, pour in the ice water slowly. Continue beating until the dough forms a ball. For an unfilled crust, prick bottom and sides and bake in a 450° oven for 10 to 12 minutes. Makes 1 crust.

Pie Crust II

2 cups barley flour
1 teaspoon salt
2/3 cup chilled leaf lard
2 tablespoons milk-free margarine,
  chilled
4 tablespoons water

If you have difficulty rolling out the dough, try patting it directly around the bottom and sides of the pie pan.

Mix together the flour and salt.

Combine the lard and margarine.

Cut half the shortening into the flour mixture with a pastry blender or work it lightly with your fingers until like cornmeal.

Cut the remaining half coarsely into the dough until it is pea size.

Sprinkle the dough with 4 tablespoons water and blend lightly into the dough. Add more water if you need to in order to gather the dough into a ball. For an unfilled crust, prick the sides and bottom of an 8-inch pie pan and bake in a 450° oven for 10 or 12 minutes.

Triple Treat

1 cup coconut milk
1/2 banana
1 teaspoon carob chips

So easy, so flexible and so delicious.

Whirl in blender. Drink.

Or, Pour into popsicle molds and freeze.

Or. Chill and eat with a spoon.

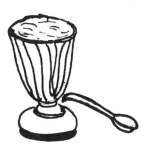

Baked Bananas

Bake bananas in their skins either in a 375° oven or an outdoor grill for about 20 minutes. Peel them and sprinkle with lemon juice or confectioners' sugar.

Poached Rhubarb

Wash and cut 1 pound of rhubarb into 1-inch pieces and place in a heavy pan. Sprinkle with water and simmer over medium heat until rhubarb can be pierced with a fork. Stir in 3/4 cup sugar and continue simmering until rhubarb is soft. Serve dusted with cinnamon or powdered ginger. Makes 4 servings.

D'Apple Rings

3 large cooking apples
(Northern Spy, Jonathan
or Winesap)
3 tablespoons milk-free margarine
confectioners' sugar
2 tablespoons water
cinnamon

Wash and core the 3 cooking apples and cut crosswise into slices.

Melt the margarine in a large skillet and place in the skillet a single layer of apple rings. Sprinkle the rings lightly with confectioners' sugar.

Add the 2 tablespoons water to the skillet, then cover and simmer until the apples are tender. Remove the cover and brown the rings on both sides. Serve sprinkled with cinnamon. Makes 4 servings.

Glazed Apples

4 cups tart apples
3 tablespoons milk-free margarine,
   melted
3/4 to 1 cup white or brown sugar

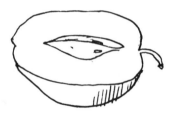

If you are ready to live dangerously, sprinkle 2 tablespoons dark rum over the apples along with the sugar.

Pare, core and thinly slice the apples.

Place them in a 6x9-inch pan and pour the melted margarine over. Bake in a 350° oven for 15 to 30 minutes until tender.

Dust with sugar and place under the broiler with the door open until the sugar glazes. Serve at once. Makes 6 servings.

Baked Pears

3 Bartlett pears
1/2 cup chopped dates
1/2 cup orange juice
1/4 cup honey
2 tablespoons milk-free margarine,
  melted
  nutmeg

Halve and core the pears and place in a baking dish. Fill the centers with dates.

Combine the orange juice, honey, and margarine and pour over the pears, then sprinkle with nutmeg.

Bake, covered, in a 350° oven for 25 minutes, basting occasionally. Makes 3 servings.

Dessert Salad

Convenient, fast, and expandable, vary this salad with what you happen to have on hand like grapes or carob chips.

Arrange avocado slices, mandarin orange segments and sliced bananas on salad greens. Sprinkle with coconut and drizzle with frozen lemonade concentrate or lime juice concentrate that has been thawed.

Riesling Berries

1 quart strawberries, hulled
1 cup raspberries
1 cup blueberries
1 to 1 1/2 cups Johannisberg Riesling

Divide berries among old fashioned champagne glasses and pour wine into each glass. Makes an elegant dessert.

Drain and wash all the berries and place them in a wide-mouthed jar. Pour the wine over and let sit for 1 hour. Makes 10 servings.

Peach Wine Dessert —Marianne Scheck

1 (3 oz.) package peach gelatin
1 (16 oz.) can sliced peaches,
  reserve 1 cup of the syrup
1 cup white wine

Follow the directions on the gelatin package, substituting the 1 cup of reserved peach syrup and the 1 cup of white wine for the water in the gelatin recipe.

Pour the gelatin mixture into sherbet glasses; cool for 20 minutes and then add the peaches. Place in refrigerator to chill. Makes 6 to 8 servings.

Arrowroot: arrowroot

Arum: poi, taro

Banana: banana

Buckwheat: buckwheat, rhubarb, garden sorrel

Caper: capers

Carrot or Parsley Family: anise, angelica, caraway seeds, carrots, celery, coriander, cumin, dill, fennel, parsley, parsnips, celeriac, celergy seed, chervil, comine, gum, galbanum, kummel, ferula gum

Chicle: chicle gum (chewing gum)

Citrus: citric acid, citron, citrange, grapefruit, kumquat, lemon, lime, orange, tangerine, tangelo

Coca: cocaine

Coffee: coffee, royoc, Indià mulberry

Cola Nut: cola nut, kutira gum

Composite or Thistle: globe artichoke, burdock, camomile, chicory, dandelion, endive, escarole, head lettuce (iceberg), safflower oil, salsify, tarragon, yarrow, boneset tea, oyster plant, feverfew, wormwort, lavender cotton, Jerusalem artichoke, sunflower seed, sunflower oil

Crustacean: crab, crayfish, lobster, shrimp

Ebony: date plum, persimmon

Fungi: moldy cheeses, mushroom, yeast

Ginger: ginger, tumeric, cardomon, arrowroot

Gooseberry: beets, beet sugar, spinach, Swiss chard

Gourd: pumpkin, squash, cucumber, cantaloupe, muskmelon, honey dew, Persian melon, casaba, watermelon, curuba, cristman melon, cassabanana, Spanish melon, zucchini

GRAINS

Barley: malt, whiskey, ale, lager, some liqueurs

Corn: hominy, corn oil, corn starch, corn syrup, dextrose, glucose, bourbon

Oat: oat flour, oatmeal

Rice: rice, wild rice

Rye: rye

Wheat: bran, gluten flours, graham flour, wheat germ, cake flour, all purpose flour, bamboo shoots, pumpernickel

Grape: cream of tartar, grape, raisin, brandy, port, sherry, wine, champagne, wine vinegar

Heath: cranberry, blueberry, huckleberry, wintergreen, bearberry

Honey: honey, bee nectar, beeswax

Honeysuckle: elderberry

Iris: saffron

Laurel: avocado, cinnamon, cassia, bay leaves, camphor, sassafras, laurel

Legume: gum arabic, kidney bean, lima bean, navy bean, soy bean (soy flour and soy oil), wax bean, locust bean gum, carob, cassia, licorice, black-eyed peas, chick peas, green peas, split peas, peanut oil, peanuts, karaya, tamarind, alfalfa, tragacanth gum

Lily: aloe, asparagus, chives, garlic, leeks, onions, sarsparilla, shallot

Macadamia Nut: Macadamia nut, Queensland nut

Mallow: okra, althea root tea, cottonseed oil, cottonseed meal, cottonseed flour

MAMMALS AND BIRDS

Cow: beef, veal, cow's milk, butter, cheese, gelatin

Goat: goat's milk, cheese

Pig: ham, pork, bacon

Sheep: mutton, lamb

Bird: chicken and eggs, duck and eggs, goose and eggs, turkey, guinea hen, squab, pheasant, partridge, grouse

Maple: maple syrup, maple sugar

Mint: mint, peppermint, spearmint, thyme, sage, marjoram, savory, pennyroyal tea, chinese artichoke, catnip, menthol, basil, bergamot, rosemary, horehound, oregano

Morning Glory: sweet potato, yam

Mulberry: breadfruit, fig, mulberry

Mullosks: abalone, mussel, oyster, scallop, clam, squid

Mustard: mustard, cabbage, cauliflower, broccoli, Brussels sprouts, turnip, rutabaga, kale, collard, celery cabbage, kohlrabi, radish, horseradish, watercress, celery cabbage, chinese cabbage, collards, sea kale, pepper grass, pepper cress, mustard green

Myrtle: allspice, cloves, pimento, paprika, guava, bayberry

Nightshade: cayenne pepper, green peppers, red peppers, eggplant, tomato, potato, tobacco, chili pepper, banana pepper, bell pepper, paprika, pimento, tabasco

Nutmeg: nutmeg, mace

NUTS

Beech: chestnut, beechnut

Birch: filbert, hazelnut, oil of birch, (perfume, winter green)

Brazil Nut: Brazil nut

Cashew: cashew, pistachio, mango

Olive: green olive, black olive, olive oil

Orchid: vanilla

Palm: cocoanut oil, cocoanut, date, sago, palm, cabbage

Pedalium: sesame oil

Pepper: black pepper, white pepper, peppercorns
Pineapple: pineapple
Pomegranate: pomegranate
Poppy: poppy seed
Potato: See Nightshade

ROSE

Rose: strawberry
Rose Family Subgroupings
Apple: apple, crabapple
Berry: blackberry, boysenberry, dewberry, loganberry, raspberry, youngberry
Pear: pear
Plum: plum, prune, cherry, peach, apricot, nectarine, almond, sloe berry (sloe gin)
Quince: quince (pectin)
Seaweed: kelp, Irish Moss (laxatives, toothpaste)
Sesame: sesame seed, sesame oil
Spurge: Jassava meal, tapioca, castor bean
Stercula: chocolate, cocoa, cocoa butter, cola beans

TEAS

Tea: green tea, black tea
Borage: comfrey tea
Buckthorn: buckthorn tea
Elm: slippery elm tea
Gentian: gentian tea
Hypericum: St. John's wort tea
Linden: linden tea
Ruta: rutin tea
Walnut: English walnut, black walnut, hickory nut, pecan, butter-nut
Water Chestnut: ling nut
(Chinese Water Chestnuts: Chinese water chestnuts)

The cross-reactivity among foods within certain families of food groupings is very strong (for example, the nightshade family and the crustacean family) and that in other food families, individuals may be sensitive to one or two foods or to none at all.

Index

Cherried Ham 50
Ham a la Orange 50
Ham Apple Ole 50
Ham with Fruit Juice
  or Sherry 50
Ham Slices Variety 50
Peachy Ham 50
Pineapple Ham 50

PORK

Gingered Pork Crown 43
Glaze 'n Spice Pork 44
Pears and Pork Chops 47
Pork Chops Pacific 46
Pork L'Orange 48
Tangy Pork Chops 45

LAMB

Festive Leg o' Lamb 37
Garlic Lamb Chops 39
Herbed Lamb Chops 39

Herbed Lamb Roll 41
Honey-Lime Lamb Roast 38
Lamb Francais 36
Lamb Shoulder Roast 42
Oranged Lamb Chops 40

VEAL

Veal Compagna 34
Veal Flambe 33
Veal Scallopini 35

POULTRY

CHICKEN

Apricot Chicken 56
Artichoke Chicken 53
Basic Chicken Stock 3
Chicken Breasts Marsala 64
Chicken Elegante 69
Chicken in the Pot 62
Chicken Limon 54
Chicken Pot Pie 65

Chicken Saute Herbed 55
Chicken Scallopini, Vin 67
Chicken Sherry 68
Lime Chicken 57
Orange Chicken 60
Pan Gravy—Poultry 70
Peach and Lime Chicken 59
Poulet Flambe 61
Poulet Marsala 63
Variety Chicken 66
Vegetable, Chicken Bake 58

TURKEY

Turkey Almondine 73
Turkey Breasts Marsala 72
Turkey Fricassee 74

CORNISH GAME HEN

Cornish Game Hen 71
Two Sauces for
  Cornish Game Hen 71

DESSERTS

Baked Bananas 182
Baked Pears 185
D'Apple Rings 183
Dessert Salad 185
Glazed Apples 184
Peach-Wine Dessert 186
Poached Rhubarb 182
Riesling Berries 186
Triple Treat 181

DRESSINGS

Apple Dressing 172
Apple-Raisin Dressing 171
Favorite Stuffing 169
Water Chestnut Stuffing 170
Wild Rice Dressing 172

GLAZES

Brown Sugar 175
Carob Glaze 136
Coffee Glaze 178
Honey Glaze 176
Honey Glaze II 178
Lemon Glaze 123
Marmalade 175
Pineapple 175

MARINADES

Herb Marinade 173
Wine Marinade 173

SAUCES

Carob Sauce 135
Cranberry Sauce 174
Lime Butter 90
Raisin Sauce 174

TOPPINGS

Caramel Topping 176
Streusel 177

MISCELLANEOUS

Pie Crust I 179
Pie Crust II 180
Strawberry Jam 37

For further information

ALLERGY INFORMATION ASSOCIATION
25 Poynter Drive, Room 7
Weston, Ontario M9R 1K8 Canada
Quarterly newsletter and various publications

AMERICAN ALLERGY ASSOCIATION
P. O. Box 7273
Menlo Park, CA 94025
Bimonthly newsletter and various publications

AMERICAN DIETETIC ASSOCIATION
430 North Michigan Avenue
Chicago, IL 60611

ASTHMA AND ALLERGY FOUNDATION OF AMERICA
9604 Wisconsin Avenue, Suite 100
Bethesda, MD 20814

THE ALLERGY BAKER
by Carol Rudoff, President, American Allergy Association
Foreword by Vincent Marinkovich, MD,
Clinical Assistant Professor of Pediatrics, Stanford University
Recipes in THE ALLERGY BAKER are free of wheat, milk, corn, soy, yeast

THE ALLERGY BAKER has a large selection of breads, cakes, cookies and muffins that have all the flavor and appeal of standard baked products. Some of the fondest memories of childhood are intertwined with the warm oven aromas of baking in the kitchen. THE ALLERGY BAKER will enable families to keep the tradition of fresh from-the-oven treats and to bake their ways to new traditions.

Send $7.95 (includes shipping) for each copy of THE ALLERGY BAKER you wish to:
PROLOGUE PUBLICATIONS
P. O. Box 640
Menlo Park, CA 94025
If you live in California, add $ .47 sales tax and mail your check for $8.42.

AMERICAN ALLERGY ASSOCIATION
P. O. Box 7273
Menlo Park, CA 94025
publishes a bimonthly newsletter, LIVING WITH ALLERGIES, to enable you to develop a better understanding of the problems of allergy and to cope with your own problems in a more knowledgeable way.
You can receive LIVING WITH ALLERGIES for a donation of $15.